# HEMODYNAMIC MONITORING
## IN CRITICAL CARE

# Contributors

**Carolyn B. Chalkey, R.N., M.S.N.**
Advanced Clinical Practice and
  Research Specialist
American Medical International—
  Brookwood Medical Center
Birmingham, Alabama
Assistant Clinical Professor, Division
  of Nursing
Birmingham Southern College

**Reba Felks-McVay, R.N., M.S.N.**
University of Alabama Hospital
Department of Nursing
Birmingham, Alabama

**Judy Dixon Fox, R.N., M.S.N.**
Coordinator, Critical Care Inservice
  Department
Carraway Methodist Medical Center
Birmingham, Alabama

**Charmaine Frederick, R.N.,
B.S.N., C.C.R.N.**
Head Nurse, Intensive Care Unit
Orlando Regional Medical Center
Orlando, Florida

**Linda J. Miers, R.N., M.S.N.**
Assistant Professor, Cardiovascular
  Nursing
University of Alabama in
  Birmingham
School of Nursing
Birmingham, Alabama

**Nancy Reeder, R.N., M.S.N.,
C.C.R.N.**
Patient Care Coordinator
Coronary Care Unit
Baptist Medical Center Montclair
Birmingham, Alabama

**Jeannie Tharpe Sizemore, R.N.,
M.S.N.**
C V Medical Clinical Nurse Specialist
Baptist Medical Center Montclair
Birmingham, Alabama

**Linda Gray Wofford, R.N.,
M.S.N., P.N.P.-C**
Instructor and Clinical Coordinator
Pediatric Nurse Practitioner Program
  at University of Virginia
Charlottesville, Virginia

**Laura C. Young, R.N., M.S.N.**
Assistant Administrator, Nursing
Bay Medical Center
Panama City, Florida

# HEMODYNAMIC MONITORING
## IN CRITICAL CARE

Edited by

### Mary Stone Price, RN, MSN
Assistant Director—Clinical
Special Care Unit
Department of Nursing
St. Thomas Hospital
Nashville, Tennessee

### Judy Dixon Fox, RN, MSN
Coordinator
Critical Care Inservice Department
Carraway Methodist Medical Center
Birmingham, Alabama

AN ASPEN PUBLICATION®
Aspen Publishers, Inc.

1987

Rockville, Maryland
Royal Tunbridge Wells

Library of Congress Cataloging-in-Publication Data

Hemodynamic monitoring in critical care.

"An Aspen publication."
Includes bibliographies and index.
1. Intraveneous catheterization. 2. Hemodynamics. 3. Patient monitoring. 4. Intensive care nursing.
5. Cardiovascular disease nursing. I. Price, Mary Stone. II. Fox, Judy Dixon. [DNLM: 1. Critical
Care — nurses' instruction. 2. Hemodynamics — nurses' instruction. 3. Monitoring,
Physiologic — methods — nurses' instruction. WG 106 H4875]
RC683.5.I5H46        1987        616'.028        86–26450
ISBN: 0–87189–398–3

Editorial Services: Carolyn Ormes

Library of Congress Catalog Card Number 86-26450
ISBN: 0-87189-398-3

*Printed in the United States of America*

1   2   3   4   5

# Contents

v

# Preface

Experienced critical care nurses who use bedside hemodynamic monitoring to assess patient conditions and determine patient management need advanced levels of knowledge to function safely in their role. Nursing foci that pertain to these patients fall into two broad categories: technical skills and critical thinking skills. Nursing integrates these two skill areas through the processes of assessing, diagnosing, planning, implementing, and evaluating patient care. Whether the experienced nurse acts as a staff nurse, preceptor, in-service instructor, or clinical nursing specialist, the need to translate theory effectively into clinical practice remains a challenge.

*Hemodynamic Monitoring in Critical Care* addresses this challenge. It is divided into two sections. Part I, Principles of Invasive Hemodynamic Monitoring, contains an extensive review of the anatomy and physiology of the cardiopulmonary system, as well as descriptions of the direct and derived parameters most commonly used in bedside hemodynamic monitoring. Principles for interpreting parameters individually and collectively are presented, and the application of these principles to selected clinical conditions is illustrated.

In Part II, Case Studies, the focus is on six cases. Included in each discussion are the use of hemodynamic parameters in that patient population, pertinent research findings, and a sample care plan. The patient populations covered by the case studies are those who have experienced multiple trauma, cardiac transplantation, sepsis, adult respiratory distress syndrome, and cardiac surgery following acute myocardial infarction. In addition, there is a single case study of a pediatric patient.

The appendixes are included as tools for those clinical nurses with expanded roles that may involve the development of standards of practice or related guidelines (e.g., policies and procedures, performance evaluations, or skills checklists), or the evaluation and/or purchase of monitoring equipment.

We would like to recognize the perseverance par excellence of each contributing author. Much time and critical thinking have been combined to bring this project to completion. Appreciation is an understatement of our feeling for the typists involved—Annie and Rita. A special note of thanks to Kathy Osten and Kathy Burns for editorial assistance with Appendix D. Lastly and most deeply, our thanks to our families and friends for the loving support that generated our creativity and courage both to begin and to finish.

# Part I

# Principles of Invasive Hemodynamic Monitoring

# Chapter 1

# The Physiologic Basis for Invasive Monitoring

*Linda J. Miers, R.N., M.S.N.*

The function of the heart is often surrounded by myth and mysticism. The heart is merely a muscular pump that propels blood to the various tissues throughout the body via the vascular system, however. Clinicians monitor the function of the heart and the flow of blood, or hemodynamics, by a variety of invasive and noninvasive techniques. In order to assess or evaluate observations and measurements fully, it is necessary to develop a thorough understanding of the heart's design and its physiologic operation.

## ANATOMY

As a muscular pump, the heart is composed of four chambers and four valves; it is connected to the vascular system by four great vessels. The two upper chambers are the atria, and the two lower chambers are the ventricles. The atria and the ventricles are divided into left and right chambers by the interatrial septum and the interventricular septum, respectively (Figure 1–1). The tricuspid valve separates the right atrium from the right ventricle, and the mitral valve separates the left atrium from the left ventricle. Between the right ventricle and the pulmonary artery lies the pulmonic valve. The aortic valve is situated between the ascending portion of the aorta and the left ventricle. The inferior and superior venae cavae drain systemic blood into the right atrium. Blood from the lungs drains into the left atrium via four pulmonary veins. There are no true valves at the outlets of the venae cavae or the pulmonary veins.

### Cardiac Cells

The muscle cells of the heart are especially designed to contract and relax in a way that moves blood from the heart to the pulmonary and systemic vessels. Other

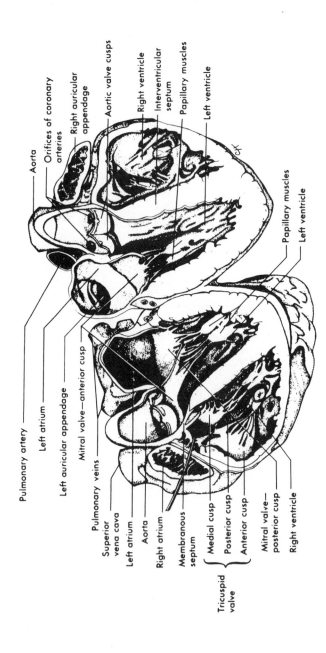

**Figure 1–1** The heart, shown split along the interventricular septum in order to illustrate the anatomical relationships of structural components.

*Source:* Reproduced by permission from *Cardiovascular Physiology*, 4th ed., by R.M. Berne and M.N. Levy, p. 85, The C.V. Mosby Company, St. Louis, © 1981.

cells are designed to permit swift conduction of the electrical impulses throughout the heart. Four cell types warrant special mention:

1. The working myocardial cells of the atria and ventricles are designed for contraction.
2. The Purkinje fibers allow rapid conduction of electrical impulses through the heart.
3. The cells found in the sinoatrial and atrioventricular nodes function as pacemakers and conduct impulses, respectively; they contain very few contractile filaments.
4. Transition cells, found in both the atria and ventricles, have an appearance somewhere between that of the Purkinje fibers and that of the working cells.

All the cells together make up a branched network of cells that is similar to, yet different from, both smooth muscle and skeletal muscle systems.

The cardiac cell contains a centrally located nucleus surrounded by a proteinaceous fluid called sarcoplasm. It also contains vast numbers of mitochondria and myofibrils. Around the cell is a membrane, known as the outer sarcolemma, that comprises a surface membrane and an outer basement membrane. At the end of each cell is the intercalated disk that connects the sarcolemma from one cell to the next and permits linear transmission of impulses from one cell to the other. There are two intracellular membrane systems, the transverse tubular system (i.e., T-tubule system) and the sarcoplasmic reticulum. The T-tubule system opens to the extracellular space and runs both transversely and longitudinally along the contractile units of the cell. The sarcoplasmic reticulum is a network of intracellular tubules, called the sarcotubular network, and surrounds the contractile proteins.

The contractile unit of the myocardial working cells is known as the sarcomere (Figure 1–2). Contractile proteins are arranged in a regular array of thick and thin filaments. The A band represents the region of the sarcomere occupied by the thick filaments into which thin filaments extend from either side. The I band is the region of the sarcomere occupied only by thin filaments; these extend toward the center of the sarcomere from the Z lines, which bisect each I band. The sarcomere is the region between each pair of Z lines; it contains two half I bands and one A band. The sarcoplasmic reticulum consists of the sarcotubular network at the center of the sarcomere and the cisternae, which abut the T-tubule system and the sarcolemma.

There are numerous sarcomeres in each cell, and they are organized in a parallel fashion along the long axis of the cell. Between the Z bands that mark adjacent sarcomere connections are many protein myofilaments, myosin and actin, that run longitudinally (Figure 1–3). The thick filaments are composed primarily of myosin molecules. The long "tails" of the myosin are parallel and form the backbone

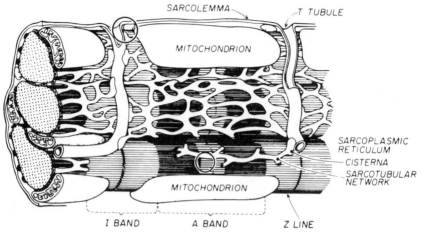

**Figure 1–2** Ultrastructure of the working myocardial cell.

*Source:* Reprinted by permission of the *New England Journal of Medicine*, Vol. 293, p. 1184, © 1975.

of the thick filament; the heads protrude at regular intervals. These myosin filaments are double-ended and have a nodular thickening at their center. Projecting from the long axes of the myosin filaments are cross-bridges that extend toward the nearby thin filaments, which are formed by molecules of actin. Threaded along the surface of these actin molecules are strands of tropomyosin; at one end of each tropomyosin strand is a molecule of troponin.

The myofibrils are composed of thick myosin filaments and thin actin filaments that generally overlap (Figure 1–4). The actin filaments are attached to the Z bands, but the myosin filaments do not extend to the Z bands. Therefore, there is an area along the Z band where the two myofilaments do not overlap—the I band. In addition, the myosin and actin filaments do not overlap at the center of the A band; this area constitutes the H zone of the A band. The amount of overlap is diminished during stretching and increased during contraction. The many cross-bridges observed at regular intervals between the actin and myosin filaments have been perceived as linkages that draw specific sites on the actin fibers onward during contraction.

The cells of the heart's conduction system differ from those of the working cells. Because they contain fewer mitochondria and myofibrils but more glycogen, they are better suited for anaerobic rather than oxidative metabolism.

## Cardiac Wall

The walls of the cardiac chambers are composed of three layers: the endocardium, the myocardium, and the epicardium. The endocardium, the internal layer,

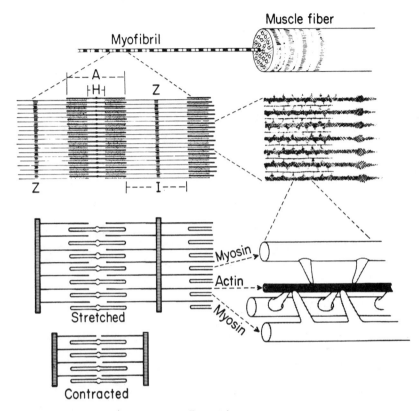

**Figure 1–3** Organization of the contractile proteins.

*Source:* Reprinted from *Cardiac Nursing* by S.L. Underhill et al., p. 16, with permission of J.B. Lippincott Company, © 1982.

---

is a thin lining of connective tissue that covers all the inner structures of the heart. The myocardium, the middle layer, is the muscular portion of the heart. The epicardium is the outer layer. Like the endocardium, it is made up of connective tissue; it is the visceral pericardium.

The heart is surrounded by a thin fibrous sac known as the pericardium. Its inner surface has already been identified as the epicardium or visceral pericardium. The outer surface, the parietal pericardium, is separated from the epicardium by a thin layer of clear fluid. This pericardial fluid, of which there is normally only 10 to 20 ml, lubricates the contracting surfaces and allows the heart to move freely within the parietal pericardium.[1] The pericardium is attached anteriorly to the sternum and posteriorly to the vertebral column. Superiorly, it is connected to the great vessels as they enter or leave the heart. Inferiorly, the pericardium is attached to the central tendon of the diaphragm.

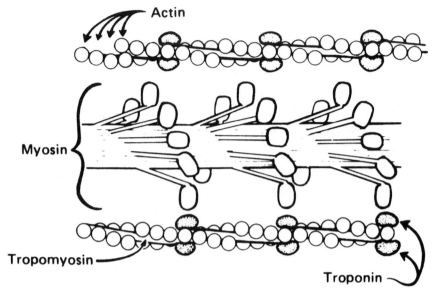

**Figure 1–4** Muscular contraction.

*Source:* Reprinted from *Structure and Function of the Cardiovascular System* by R.F. Rushmer, p. 81, with permission of the W.B. Saunders Company, © 1976.

While the pericardium is functionally useful in that it contains the heart and defines the upper limit to which the heart is able to enlarge, it is not essential. Moreover, this inelastic confinement by the pericardium may restrict the contractile function of the heart if the heart enlarges excessively or if the sac fills with an abundance of fluid. If the pericardium is congenitally absent or surgically removed, the heart appears to function within its physiologic limits.

### Cardiac Valves

The basic structures of the heart's valves are the fibrous valve ring (i.e., the annulus) and the valve leaflets. The leaflets are thin, flexible structures of endothelium-covered fibrous tissue that are tough enough to withstand the wear and tear produced by 80 or so years of continuous blood flow, high pressure, and repetitive opening and closing. The movement of the valve leaflets is essentially a passive response to pressure gradients, and the design of the leaflets is such that they guide the flow of blood unidirectionally through the heart. There are two types of valves, the atrioventricular and the semilunar, in the heart (see Figure 1–1; Figure 1–5).

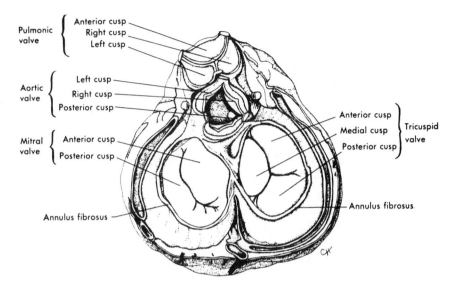

**Figure 1–5** The four cardiac valves viewed from the base of the heart. Note the manner in which the leaflets overlap in the closed valves.

*Source:* Reproduced by permission from *Cardiovascular Physiology*, 4th ed., by R.M. Berne and M.N. Levy, p. 85, The C.V. Mosby Company, St. Louis, © 1981.

*Atrioventricular Valves*

The two atrioventricular valves, identified earlier as the tricuspid and mitral valves, are larger and have a more complex structure than do the semilunar valves. Each atrioventricular valve has six components:

1. the atrium
2. the fibrous valve ring, or annulus
3. the valvular leaflets
4. the chordae tendineae
5. the papillary muscles
6. the ventricular wall

The complicated interaction of these components influences the flow of blood from the atria to the ventricles. Dysfunction of any one of these components can have serious hemodynamic consequences.

Anatomically, the tricuspid and mitral valves are fundamentally the same, even though the former appears to have three leaflets (i.e., cusps) and the latter appears to have two (see Figure 1–5). The leaflets are identified according to their location and their relationship to surrounding structures. The chordae tendineae, small tendinous cords of collagen strands that often subdivide and interconnect, may attach anywhere along the free edge or even a few millimeters back from the edge of the leaflet. They extend inferiorly to the papillary muscles. The chordae tendineae of the tricuspid valve usually attach to an adjacent anterior, posterior, or septal (medial) papillary muscle in the right ventricle, although some may attach directly to the adjacent ventricular wall. The chordae tendineae of the mitral valve attach to an adjacent anterior or posterior papillary muscle, or directly to the adjacent left ventricular myocardial wall. Dysfunction of a papillary muscle or rupture of a chorda tendinea may weaken the support of the valve leaflets, leading to regurgitation.

The orifice of the tricuspid valve, greater than 7 $cm^2$, is larger than that of the mitral valve, and it has a semivertical axis.[2] It directs blood from the right atrium anteriorly, inferiorly, and to the left. Its leaflets are thinner, more translucent, and less easily separated into distinct leaflets than are those of the mitral valve. The anterior leaflet, which is the largest, is followed in size by the septal leaflet (medial cusp). The posterior leaflet is usually the smallest.

The mitral valve orifice is usually 4 to 6 $cm^2$ and faces anterolaterally, thus directing blood from the left atrium anteriorly, inferiorly, and leftward.[3] The two major leaflets, the anteromedial and the posterolateral, are linked by commissural tissue. The anteromedial leaflet, more commonly known as the anterior leaflet, is continuous with supporting tissues of the noncoronary and left coronary aortic cusps. The ventricular surface of the anterior leaflet forms the posterosuperior portion of the left ventricular outflow tract. The posterolateral leaflet, generally known as the posterior leaflet (cusp), is longer and less mobile than the anterior one and encircles two-thirds of the circumference of the mitral valve orifice.

*Semilunar Valves*

The valves that separate the pulmonary artery and the aorta from their associated ventricles, the pulmonic and aortic valves respectively, are known as the semilunar valves (see Figures 1-1 and 1-5). They are structurally similar, although the aortic valve cusps are slightly thicker than are the pulmonic valve cusps to accommodate the higher pressures of the left ventricle. Each valve is a three-cusp structure in which the cusps are arranged to encircle the root of the vessel. The lower edges of the cusps are attached to and suspended from the root of the associated great vessel; the upper free edges project into the lumen of the vessel. The vessel wall bulges behind each cusp, forming a pouch or pocketlike dilation that is called the sinus of Valsalva. The design of the valve cusps and the strong fibrous support allow for adequate closure of the leaflets during diastole, thus preventing regurgitation of blood, and for passive opening during systole, thus permitting ejection of blood to the lungs or periphery.

The leaflets or cusps of each semilunar valve are identified either by their location or, in the case of the aortic valve, by their relationship to the coronary arteries. The pulmonic cusps are called anterior, right, and left; the aortic cusps are called right coronary, left coronary, and noncoronary cusps. The right and left coronary cusps are anterior structures, whereas the noncoronary cusp is posterior. The openings, or ostia, of the coronary arteries are located in the upper third of the sinus of Valsalva.

## Cardiac Chambers and Great Vessels

Blood returns from the periphery to the heart via the venous system. Specifically, blood returns to the right atrium from the large venous vessels known as the venae cavae. The superior vena cava empties blood from the head and upper extremities, whereas the inferior vena cava drains blood from the abdomen and lower extremities. Although there are no formal valve structures to separate these vessels from the right atrium, there is a slight pressure gradient between the venae cavae and the right atrium that aids in venous return to the heart.

### Right Heart Chambers

Positioned above, behind, and to the right of the right ventricle, the right atrium forms the right lateral cardiac border. It is anterior and to the right of the left atrium. The right atrial inner surface is smooth on the posterior and medial (i.e., septal) walls, but the surfaces of the lateral wall and the atrial appendage are made up of parallel muscle bundles. The wall of the right atrium is approximately 2 mm thick. The atrial septum is located in the posteroinferior portion of the right atrium's medial wall and continues diagonally forward from right to left. The fossa ovalis, a shallow depression near the center of the interatrial septum, is the remnant of the embryonic foramen ovale.[4]

Blood from the right atrium passes through the tricuspid valve into the right ventricle, which then propels that blood into the pulmonary vasculature. The right ventricle is situated anteriorly and lies just beneath the sternum. It is positioned below, in front of, and medial to the right atrium, anterior and to the right of the left ventricle. The right ventricle is a crescent-shaped chamber whose outer wall is 4 to 5 mm thick.[5] The interventricular septum, which serves as the medial wall of both ventricles, protrudes into the right ventricular cavity, contributing to the chamber's crescent shape as the anterior right ventricular wall curves over it. The anterior and inferior walls of the right ventricle are covered by muscle bundles, known as the trabeculae carneae, that generally form ridges along the wall surface or cross from one wall to the other. One constant muscle bundle, the moderator band, extends from the lower ventricular septum across to the anterior wall and joins the anterior papillary muscle.

The right ventricle can be divided into two tracts, the inflow tract and the outflow tract. The inflow tract comprises the tricuspid valve and the trabecular muscles of the anterior and inferior walls. In this tract, blood flows from the atrium anteriorly, inferiorly, and to the left at a 60° angle to the outflow tract.[6] The smooth-walled outflow tract, also known as the infundibulum, forms the superior portion of the right ventricle. A thick muscle band, the crista supraventricularis, separates the inflow tract from the outflow tract as it arches from the anterolateral wall to the septal wall. Blood that enters the outflow tract is directed superiorly and posteriorly into the pulmonary artery.

*Pulmonary Vasculature*

The primary functions of the pulmonary circulation are the uptake of oxygen and the release of carbon dioxide by the blood. So that these processes can occur as efficiently and effectively as possible, the pulmonary circulatory system differs from the systemic circulatory system in a number of ways. Although the main pulmonary artery closely resembles the aorta in design, the pulmonary vessels are shorter and wider than are comparable systemic vessels. The arterial walls of the pulmonary vascular network are thinner and possess little or no contractile tissue at the capillary level. The capillary network within the lung is extremely dense around the many alveoli in order to promote rapid diffusion of gases.

The lungs have a secondary circulatory system, the bronchial arteries. These arteries supply oxygenated blood to the walls of the bronchial network, including the bronchioles; to the supporting tissue of the lungs; to the pulmonary nerves and sensory endings; and to the small vessels that supply the larger pulmonary arteries. Only about 1 percent of the right ventricular cardiac output is transmitted to the bronchial arteries. The bronchial venous outflow is discharged into the pulmonary veins. Generally, this venous drainage into the oxygenated flow of the pulmonary veins does not present a problem. When pulmonary flow is decreased to one or both lungs, however, bronchial flow may be increased; this increase may result in a significant venous shunt and arterial desaturation.

The pulmonary veins, of which there are four, enter the posterolateral walls of the left atrium. Even though there are no valves at the end of the pulmonary veins, extensions of atrial muscle form a sleevelike structure around the pulmonary veins for 1 to 2 cm. They may exert a sphincterlike effect, thus decreasing the amount of reflux during atrial systole or mitral regurgitation.[7]

*Left Heart Chambers*

The left atrium receives oxygenated blood from the pulmonary veins. During ventricular systole, it serves as a holding chamber; during ventricular diastole, as a channel for flow. The left atrium is positioned superiorly, medially, and posteriorly to other cardiac chambers. The esophagus rests just beneath its posterior surface, and the root of the aorta encroaches on its anterior wall. With a thickness of 3 mm, the wall of the left atrium is slightly thicker than that of the right atrium.[8] The endocardium of this chamber is smooth and slightly opaque. The septal wall of the left atrium is also smooth, and similar to its right atrial counterpart, it may exhibit a shallow central area that corresponds to the fossa ovalis. Only in the left atrial appendage, which extends from the anterolateral left atrium and along the pulmonary artery, are pectinate muscles, or muscle bands, found in the left atrium.

The left ventricle receives blood from the left atrium via the mitral valve during ventricular diastole and ejects blood to the aorta and systemic circulatory network during ventricular systole. Generally, the left ventricle is cone-shaped with a blunt tip that is directed anteriorly, inferiorly, and to the left. The major portion of the external surface of the left ventricle is posterior and to the left of the right ventricle, and inferior, anterior, and to the left of the left atrium. The muscular walls of this chamber measure 8 to 15 mm, except at the tip of the apex where the wall is thinner, measuring 2 mm or less.[9] As mentioned earlier, the interventricular septum, a generally triangular structure, serves as the medial surface of both ventricles; functionally, however, it resembles the free wall of the left ventricle. The septum is almost entirely muscular, except for the small membranous portion that is located just below the right coronary and posterior cusps of the aortic valve. The upper one-third of the septum is smooth endocardium, while the lower two-thirds and the remaining ventricular walls are lined with trabeculae carneae.

Like the right ventricle, the left ventricle can be separated into an inflow and an outflow tract. The inflow tract, which is funnel-shaped, is created by the mitral annulus, both mitral leaflets, and the chordae tendineae. Blood is directed inferiorly, anteriorly, and to the left. The outflow tract is formed by the inferior surface of the anteromedial leaflet of the mitral valve, the ventricular septum, and the left ventricular free wall. Blood is directed from the apex to the right and superiorly. During ventricular systole, the mitral leaflets are pushed upward into their closed position, and the entire left ventricle becomes an ejectile chamber.

## Aorta

Blood flows from the left ventricle into the aorta, which has a diameter of 2.5 cm. Through its arterial network, the aorta distributes blood to the heart and the rest of the body.[10] Like the pulmonary artery, the aorta is derived from the embryonic truncus arteriosus. At birth, the walls of these two vessels have an approximately equal thickness; in the adult, however, the walls of the aorta are much thicker than are those of the pulmonary artery. The walls of the aorta measure approximately 2 mm.[11] The large number of elastic fibers in the walls allows the aortic arch to expand and become a reservoir during ventricular ejection, as well as to contract and convert the pulsatile flow to a nearly continuous flow during the latter portion of systole and all of diastole.

### Cardiac Vasculature

The heart receives its blood supply from a rich network of arteries and arterioles that branch from two main coronary arteries. The right coronary artery arises from the right coronary sinus at the root of the aorta, while the left coronary artery arises from the upper half of the left coronary sinus of the aorta, behind the pulmonary trunk. The left coronary artery branches into two, three, or more divisions (Figures 1–6 and 1–7).

*Left Coronary Artery*

The initial portion of the left coronary artery, commonly known as the left main coronary artery, varies in length from a few millimeters to a few centimeters and lies free in epicardial fat. Generally, it is thought that the vessel bifurcates into two branches, but it is commonly found to divide into three or more equally large

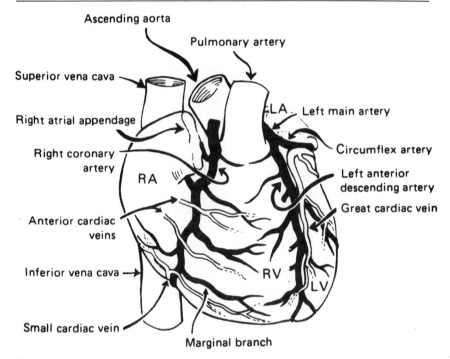

**Figure 1–6** Principal arteries and veins on the anterior surface of the heart. Part of the right atrial appendage has been resected. *RA,* right atrium; *RV,* right ventricle; *LA,* left atrium; *LV,* left ventricle.

*Source:* Reprinted from *Cardiac Nursing* by S.L. Underhill et al., p. 10, with permission of J.B. Lippincott Company, © 1982.

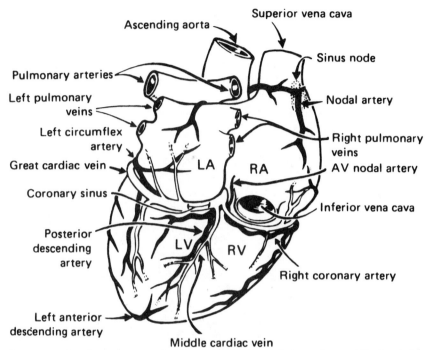

**Figure 1–7** Principal arteries and veins on the inferior-posterior surfaces of the heart. As drawn here, the heart is tilted upward at a nonphysiologic angle; normally, little of the inferior cardiac surface is visible posteriorly. The sulci are not depicted; however, the coronary sinus lies in the atrioventricular sulcus, while the middle cardiac vein and the posterior descending artery course in the interventricular sulcus. The right coronary artery is shown to cross the crux and to supply the atrioventricular node. The artery to the sinus node is depicted as arising from the right coronary artery. *RA,* right atrium; *RV,* right ventricle; *LA,* left atrium; *LV,* left ventricle; *AV,* atrioventricular.

*Source:* Reprinted from *Cardiac Nursing* by S.L. Underhill et al., p. 10, with permission of J.B. Lippincott Company, © 1982.

---

divisions. One large branch, called the left anterior descending artery, extends down the anterior surface of the heart in the groove that separates the external anterior surface of the right and left ventricles, or the interventricular sulcus. Another branch, the left circumflex artery, extends into the atrioventricular sulcus. One, two, or three other branches, commonly referred to as diagonal left ventricular branches of the main left coronary artery, are distributed diagonally over the free wall of the left ventricle. Usually, they are proportionately spaced between the anterior descending and circumflex arteries.

The left anterior descending coronary artery branches in two directions. Some branches extend over the free wall of the left ventricle, while others penetrate and curve posteriorly into the ventricular septum. Smaller branches are distributed to the nearby wall of the right ventricle. Rarely does the left anterior descending coronary artery terminate on the anterior surface of the heart; it almost always curves around to the posterior interventricular sulcus and continues 2 to 5 cm superiorly, extending branches to the posterior surfaces of the apex of the left and right ventricles.[12] At its termination point, it is met by distal branches of the posterior descending artery (see Figures 1–6 and 1–7).

The left circumflex artery typically begins at a sharp angle of 90° or more from the left main coronary artery and courses in a direction almost opposite to that of the left main artery. The initial portion of the left circumflex artery is normally covered by the left atrial appendage. It ascends into the left coronary sulcus and extends to the obtuse margin of the left ventricle, where it emerges from under the left atrial appendage and is covered by epicardial fat. At this point, it usually extends inferiorly along the left ventricle toward the apex. It provides branches to the diaphragmatic surface of the left ventricle and to the posterior interventricular sulcus, where the branches are met by terminal branches of the right coronary artery.

In only about 10 percent of humans does the left circumflex artery itself continue in the posterior portion of the atrioventricular sulcus, cross the crux of the heart (i.e., the point on the posterior surface of the heart where the atrioventricular sulci cross the interventricular sulci), and turn down the posterior interventricular sulcus to form one or more posterior descending arteries.[13] In these hearts, branches of the left coronary artery supply the whole left ventricle and interventricular septum. Branches of the left circumflex artery supply most of the left atrium and the lateral wall, as well as a portion of the posterior wall of the left ventricle. In 45 percent of human hearts, an atrial branch of the left circumflex artery supplies the sinus node.[14]

### Right Coronary Artery

Arising from the right coronary sinus of the aorta, the right coronary artery extends into the right atrioventricular sulcus, where it is covered fairly well by epicardial fat (see Figures 1–6 and 1–7). In a vast majority of humans, 90 percent, it continues to the posterior atrioventricular sulcus, crosses the crux of the heart, and divides, going on in two directions.[15] Two or more branches extend toward the apex, and another continues in the left atrioventricular sulcus to supply approximately 50 percent of the diaphragmatic surface of the left ventricle. The right ventricular branches of the right coronary artery supply the ventricle as they extend down the right edge of the heart toward the apex and anterior interventricular sulcus. In approximately 55 percent of humans, the right coronary artery supplies blood to the sinus node.[16]

*Coronary Veins*

The coronary venous system comprises three systems of veins (see Figures 1–6 and 1–7). The largest system, which drains the left ventricle, is the coronary sinus vein and its tributaries. This system begins with the anterior interventricular vein, which parallels the left anterior descending artery into the atrioventricular sulcus. At this point, it becomes the great cardiac vein and receives blood from small tributary veins from the left ventricle. Approximately halfway along this vein, where a small left atrial vein enters, the great cardiac vein becomes the coronary sinus, which continues on to its entrance into the right atrium. Where the great cardiac vein becomes the coronary sinus, a fold of endothelium forms a rudimentary valve. Several large tributary veins from various portions of the left ventricle drain into the coronary sinus, although an occasional vein drains directly into the right atrium. The opening between the coronary sinus and the right atrium is protected by the thebesian valve, an inefficient semilunar fold of endothelium.

The second venous system, which comprises the anterior cardiac veins, is intermediate in size. These veins form over the anterior wall of the right ventricle, create two or three large trunks, drain in the direction of the anterior right atrioventricular sulcus, and empty directly into the right atrium. The many anastomoses between the anterior cardiac veins and the tributaries of the coronary sinus provide alternate drainage routes in times of increased resistance in either of the two systems.

The smallest of the venous systems is that of the thebesian veins. Because these veins are quite small, the venous drainage through them is minimal. These veins are generally found in the right atrium and ventricle, but they occasionally occur on the left heart surfaces as well. In either case, they are most numerous near the septa. They drain directly into the right atrium near the orifice of the coronary sinus.

## Cardiac Conduction System

Specialized cells that initiate and conduct electrical impulses within the heart make up the cardiac conduction system. This system includes the sinus node, the internodal and interatrial pathways, the atrioventricular node, and the atrioventricular bundle and its proximal and distal branches (Figure 1–8).

The sinus node is located near the junction of the superior vena cava and the right atrium. It is approximately 10 to 20 mm long and is generally shaped like a flattened ellipse. Because the sinus node lies approximately 1 mm below the epicardium, it is very susceptible to diseases that affect the surface of the heart. Through the center of the node passes a large artery, branches of which supply the node. The artery is one of the first branches of the main right coronary artery, and it

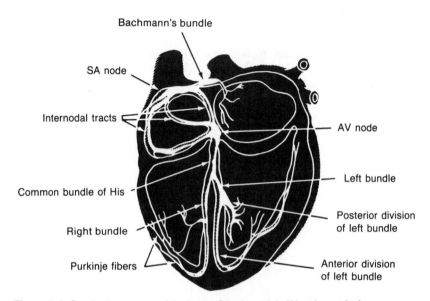

**Figure 1–8** Conduction system of the heart. *SA,* sinoatrial; *AV,* atrioventricular.

*Source:* Reproduced with permission. *Advanced Cardiac Life Support Manual,* p. IV.2, © 1975. American Heart Association.

is speculated that there is a relationship between the pressure and pulsation of the artery and the pacemaking function of the node.[17]

Within the midportion of the sinus node are an abundant number of P cells, considered the pacemaking cells of the sinus node; there are fewer of these cells at the periphery. Distributed from the cells are sinus node fibers that lie near nerve endings. There are numerous nerve endings within the node, but no ganglia. Ganglia are, however, found at the anterior and posterior edges of the node.

Extending from the sinus node are three specialized conduction pathways. They are labeled according to their anatomical origin and position as the anterior, middle, and posterior internodal pathways. They are composed of both ordinary and Purkinje fibers, but there are greater numbers of Purkinje fibers. These pathways allow rapid conduction of impulses through the right atrium to the atrioventricular node. From the anterior internodal pathway extends an interatrial pathway known as Bachmann's bundle. Even though extensions of the other internodal pathways reach into the right atrium, Bachmann's bundle appears to be the preferred interatrial pathway.

The atrioventricular node lies strategically between the atria and the ventricles. It receives fibers of the terminal portion of the internodal pathways at its anterior and posterior surface. It performs ''triage'' on the atrial impulses transmitted to the ventricles, delaying transmission of the impulses by approximately 0.04

second. This delay appears to occur at or near the atrionodal junction. Structurally, the atrioventricular node is both similar to and different from the sinus node. Like the sinus node, it contains P cells. The fibers of the atrioventricular node, however, are slightly thicker and shorter than those of the sinus node. In the upper and middle portion of the atrioventricular node, the fibers randomly interweave to form a meshlike network similar to that in the sinus node. At the anterior and inferior portions of the node, the fibers begin to take on a more longitudinal orientation. Behind the atrioventricular node are a number of autonomic ganglia, presumably vagal; together with adjacent neural structures, these ganglia may have receptor functions. Furthermore, they may be the means by which extracardiac vagal stimuli enter the atrioventricular node. Blood supply to this node is via the right coronary artery in 90 percent of human hearts.[18]

The longitudinal fibers of the atrioventricular node converge to form the parallel fibers of the atrioventricular bundle, which descends from the atrioventricular node along the posterior margin of the membranous interventricular septum to the top of the muscular septum. The atrioventricular bundle gives rise to the right and left bundle branches. As a single, slender group of fibers, the right bundle branch exits from the common bundle just below the junction of the membranous and muscular portions of the ventricular septum. The left bundle branch appears as a sheet of fibers extending from the left edge of the common bundle. The two branches extend along the endocardium in a generally anterior and apical direction, spreading out in all directions to cover the ventricular wall. Approximately 20 to 30 mm beyond the beginning of the left bundle branch, two relatively direct pathways to the anterior and posterior papillary muscles are formed.[19]

Fibers of the atrioventricular bundle are arranged in a parallel fashion. Initially larger than those of the atrioventricular node, the fibers become even larger after the bifurcation into the right and left branches and have a greater diameter than do myocardial fibers. Many of these fibers resemble the classic Purkinje fibers in structure. Others resemble those ordinarily found in the myocardium, and it has been suggested that these fibers may possess rapid conduction capabilities.

### Peripheral Vasculature

The peripheral vascular system is made up of an extensive network of arteries and veins. The arterial system is an extension of the aorta; it delivers oxygen and other nutrients to the body. In addition, the arterial network controls the flow and pressure of blood after its ejection from the left ventricle. The venous system transports carbon dioxide and other metabolic wastes back to the lungs and other organs of elimination. Furthermore, because the venous network also serves as a capacitance system, it helps to control the amount of blood returned to the heart. Between the arteries and veins are the capillaries, where gases and particulate matter are exchanged.

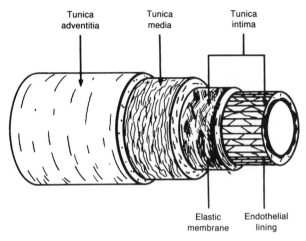

**Figure 1-9** Tissue layers of the arterial wall.

The arterial walls are composed of three layers (Figure 1–9). The inner layer is the tunica intima, which is composed of an internal elastic membrane and an endothelial lining. The middle layer, the tunica media, is composed of smooth muscle and elastic tissue. The outer layer is the tunica adventitia, which consists of collagenous and elastic tissue. The smaller the arteries, the more muscular and less elastic they are. Moreover, the walls of the larger, more elastic arteries are thinner than are those of smaller arteries (Figure 1–10).

From the arteries, blood flows to the arterioles, which are composed of an endothelial layer and a continuous layer of smooth muscle. Smaller than arteries are, they range in size from 20 to 50 μm.[20] The metarterioles found in some vascular beds are distinguished from arterioles by their size, 10 to 15 μm, and structure, a single, noncontinuous layer of smooth muscle. From the arterioles or metarterioles branch the arterial capillaries. At the junction of these two structures is the precapillary sphincter, a band of vascular smooth muscle that regulates blood flow to the capillaries and controls blood pressure by its opening and closing.

Capillaries are composed of a single layer of endothelium that is surrounded by a basement membrane on the outside. The total wall thickness is 0.5 μm.[21] Because capillaries have no smooth muscle, their resistance to blood flow is low. Some capillaries, called preferential capillaries, are larger than are the smaller, true capillaries. Arterial capillaries are generally smaller than venous capillaries, measuring 5 μm compared to 8 μm.[22] Blood flows from the venous capillaries into elastic, nonmuscular venules and then to muscular venules (Figure 1–11).

Veins are more numerous than arteries are, and they have a larger diameter and thinner walls than do their arterial counterparts. The walls of veins contain

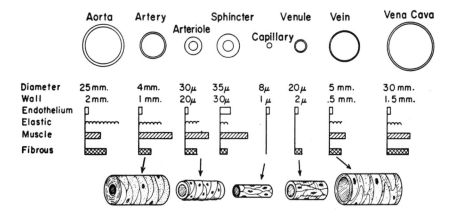

**Figure 1–10** Components of the vascular walls. The relative amounts of elastic tissue and fibrous tissue are largest in the aorta and least in small branches of the arterial tree. Smaller vessels have more prominent smooth muscle in the media. Capillaries consist only of endothelial tubes. The walls of the veins are much like the arterial walls, but they are thinner in relation to their caliber.

*Source:* Reprinted from *Structure and Function of the Cardiovascular System* by R.F. Rushmer, p. 135, with permission of W.B. Saunders Company, © 1976.

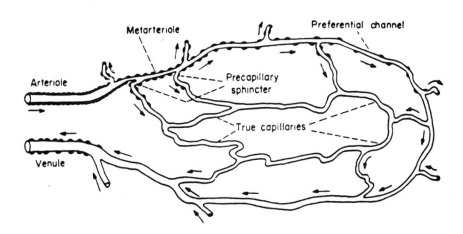

**Figure 1–11** Overall structure of a capillary bed.

*Source:* Reprinted from *Factors Regulating Blood Pressure* by B.W. Zweifach, p. 251, with permission, Josiah Macy, Jr. Foundation, © 1950.

minimal smooth muscle and are, therefore, more elastic than are the walls of arteries. Differentiation of the three muscle layers is often difficult. Deeper veins anastomose with superficial veins to form a rich venous network.

Some veins have valves that aid in returning blood to the heart. Generally greater than 1 mm in diameter, these veins are located in the neck and extremities. The valves are paired semilunar membranes of thin connective tissue and are designed to promote forward flow and to prevent retrograde flow. At the intersection of the valve and the vein wall, which is thinner at this point, there is a sinus. There are no valves in the veins of the head, thorax, or abdomen.

Innervation of the arteries and veins is both sensory and autonomic in nature. The nerves are embedded in the adventitia of the vessel wall. The arterioles and the splanchnic and cutaneous veins are richly innervated, while the metarterioles and precapillary sphincters are poorly innervated. Because capillaries are not innervated, they are not under the control of the central nervous system.

## PHYSIOLOGY

In order to propel blood throughout the body, the specially designed cells of the heart must contract and relax rhythmically. Some cells are designed to establish and conduct rhythmic electrical impulses, while others are designed to perform the mechanical work necessary to move the blood. Various mechanisms regulate both the electrical and mechanical events in order to control the amount and velocity of blood flow. The combination and interaction of these electrical, mechanical, and regulatory occurrences is essential to the effective pumping action of the heart.

### Muscle Mechanics

Contraction and relaxation of myocardial cells results from the interaction between the protein filaments actin and myosin at the site of the cross-bridges. The electrolyte essential to this interaction is calcium.

#### Electromechanics

The resting cardiac cell is polarized, that is, there is a negative electrical charge inside the cell and a positive electrical charge in the surrounding extracellular fluid. The membrane potential is the voltage difference between the interior and exterior of the cell. The sarcolemma, a semipermeable membrane, controls the electrical state of the cell through its regulation of the influx and efflux of various ions. In the resting state, for example, the cell membrane is very permeable to potassium and relatively impermeable to sodium, chloride, and calcium. Thus, potassium can easily diffuse across the membrane in response to ion gradients.

The permeability of the membrane changes in a sequential fashion, however, creating the cardiac action potential.

The cardiac action potential is comprised of four phases, numbered in order from 0 through 3 (Figure 1–12). A fifth phase, phase 4, occurs between action potentials. During phase 0, the cell depolarizes (i.e., the charge inside the cell becomes less negative). This occurs because of the rapid influx of the positive sodium ion through fast sodium channels in the cell membrane. At this time, the cell becomes relatively impermeable to potassium. At the end of this phase, the fast sodium channels close, and phase 1 begins. Known as the early repolarization phase, phase 1 exhibits a slight increase in negative potential with a rapid, but brief, influx of the negative chloride ion. The longest portion of the action potential is phase 2, or the plateau phase. During this phase, the slow influx of calcium is balanced by the slow efflux of potassium, which maintains the electrical charge of the cell at a relative steady state. At the end of this phase, the influx of calcium declines, and the cell once again becomes very permeable to potassium. Phase 3, or repolarization, begins at this point. During this phase, potassium rapidly leaves the cell, causing the cell to return to its resting potential.

At the end of phase 3, or at the end of the action potential, the ionic composition of the cell is altered in that potassium has been exchanged for sodium. The mechanism that restores the cell's original composition is the sodium pump.

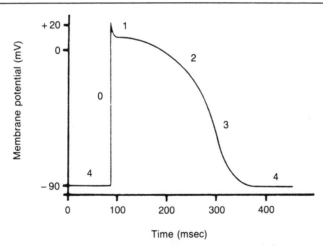

**Figure 1–12** Cardiac action potential. Shown here for a Purkinje fiber, the cardiac action potential lasts over 300 msec and consists of four phases plus resting potential. Phase 0 (upstroke) corresponds to depolarization in skeletal muscle, and phase 3 corresponds to repolarization in that tissue. Phases 1 (early repolarization) and 2 (plateau) have no clear counterpart in skeletal muscle. A fifth phase, phase 4 (diastole), corresponds to the resting potential.

*Source:* Reprinted from *Physiology of the Heart* by A.M. Katz, p. 230, with permission of Raven Press, New York, © 1977.

During phase 4, the resting potential phase, sodium is exchanged for potassium by means of an adenosine triphosphate (ATP)–dependent enzyme. This exchange requires energy, because both ions are moved against a concentration gradient. The sodium pump exchanges three sodium ions for only two potassium ions; therefore, it tends to make the electrical charges in the cell's interior more negative in comparison to that in the exterior.[23]

The action potential of cells in the heart is longer than that of cells in skeletal muscle. Moreover, because the action potential of skeletal cells has no phases, the action potential of cardiac cells is more complex. In fact, the characteristics of the action potential within the heart differ from one region to another. This is related to the differences in ionic channels of the sarcolemma for the various cardiac cell types.

*Contractile Process*

Muscles contract via a sliding filament mechanism that results from an interactive force between the actin and myosin filaments. When a muscle contracts, the thin actin filaments slide over the thicker myosin filaments, pulling the Z bands toward the ends of the myosin filaments (see Figure 1–4). When the muscle relaxes, the actin filaments slide back so that their ends barely overlap one another.

In the relaxed or resting state, the interaction of the thin and thick filaments is inhibited. It is believed that the troponin-tropomyosin complex (of the actin filament) that is not bound to calcium blocks the active site on the filament.[24] When an action potential travels over the sarcolemma, however, large quantities of calcium ions are released from the sarcoplasmic reticulum where they were stored after their influx into the cell during the previous action potential and from the T-tubule system. These calcium ions bind with the troponin molecule and inhibit the blockage of the active site. This activates the interactive forces between the filaments, and contraction begins. The energy required for the continuation of this contractile process is obtained from the degradation of ATP to adenosine diphosphate (ADP).

The interaction of actin and myosin appears to occur when the head of the myosin protrusion, or cross-bridge, couples with the active site on the actin filament. The myosin filament is composed of approximately 200 myosin molecules.[25] Each myosin molecule has two parts, a light meromyosin and a heavy meromyosin (Figure 1–13). The light meromyosin is a helix of two peptide strands. The heavy meromyosin consists of two parts: a double helix not unlike that of the light meromyosin and a head attached to the end of the double helix rod. The head is a composite of two globular protein masses. At the junction of the light and heavy meromyosin rods, the molecule is flexible and is said to have a hingelike joint. In fact, the extension of the heads is controlled by the rod portion of the heavy meromyosin, which acts as a hinged arm. There is another hinge at the

**A**

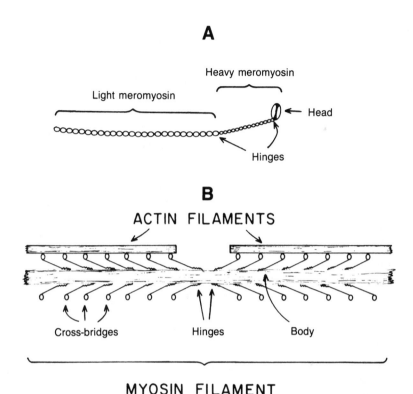

**Figure 1–13** Cardiac myofibrils. *A.* Myosin molecule. *B.* Combination of many myosin molecules, forming a myosin filament. Also shown are the cross-bridges and the interaction between the heads of the cross-bridges with adjacent actin filaments.

*Source:* Reprinted from *Textbook of Medical Physiology* by A.C. Guyton, p. 134, with permission of W.B. Saunders Company, © 1976.

juncture of the rod and the head of the heavy meromyosin. The light meromyosin strands aggregate to form the myosin filament; the heavy meromyosin rods and their heads constitute the cross-bridges. The arms of the cross-bridges extend away from the center of the filament toward the two ends.

The head of the myosin cross-bridge contains an enzyme, ATP-ase, that degrades ATP to ADP and inorganic phosphate ($P_i$). The chemical energy created by this process is converted to the mechanical energy of contraction.

The backbone of the actin filament is a double-stranded protein molecule wound in a helix. Attached to each strand of the helix is one ADP molecule, believed to be the active site with which the myosin cross-bridge interacts. As noted earlier, the actin helix also contains troponin and tropomyosin (see Figure 1–3). Troponin has a very strong affinity for calcium, which explains the binding of calcium to the troponin-tropomyosin complex that was discussed earlier.

The ratchet theory of contraction is the hypothesis used to explain the way in which the interaction between the myosin cross-bridges and actin causes contraction (Figure 1–14).[26] The cross-bridge heads attach to and detach from the active sites of the actin filament. When this attachment occurs, the hinge at the juncture of the head and the rod becomes flexible, allowing the head to tilt toward the center of the myosin filament. As it tilts, it drags the actin filament with it. This head tilt is called a power stroke.[27] After tilting, the head automatically splits from the actin's active site, returns to its former upright position, attaches to a new active site, and creates another power stroke. In this step-by-step fashion, the heads of the myosin cross-bridges pull the actin filaments toward the center of the myosin filament, using the active sites as cogs of a ratchet. Contraction continues as long as the concentration of calcium is great enough to maintain it.

The muscle relaxes when the T-tubules and the sarcolemma repolarize and the calcium concentration in the vicinity of the troponin-tropomyosin complex decreases below a critical level. This depletion in calcium concentration results from the active uptake of calcium by the sarcoplasmic reticulum, the use of calcium by the mitochondria, and the active pumping of calcium out of the cell through the walls of the T-tubule. In effect, the duration of contraction is directly related to the length of the action potential, that is, approximately 150 msec in atrial muscle and 300 msec in ventricular muscle.[28]

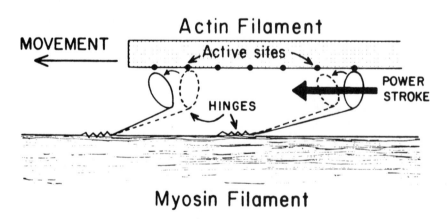

**Figure 1–14** Ratchet mechanism for contraction of the muscle.

*Source:* Reprinted from *Textbook of Medical Physiology* by A.C. Guyton, p. 136, with permission of W.B. Saunders Company, © 1976.

## Cardiac Cycle

In order to act as a pump, the heart must fill and empty in a rhythmic fashion. The period of time when the cardiac muscle fibers are relaxed and the chambers are filling with blood is called diastole. Systole is the period when the muscles are contracting and blood is ejected from the chambers. One cardiac cycle is the combination of diastole and systole, or from the end of one contraction to the end of the next (Figure 1–15).

### Electrical Events

In the normal cardiac cycle, electrical events establish the rate and rhythm for the mechanical events so that the atria contract before the ventricles contract. The complete electrical cycle consists of a P, Q, R, S, and T wave.

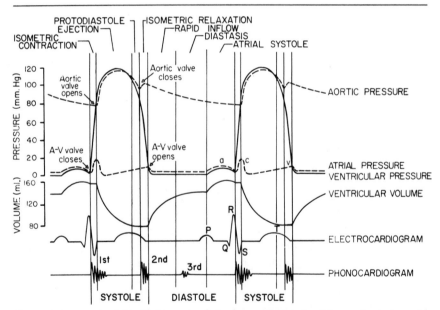

**Figure 1–15** Events of the cardiac cycle. At the top are the labels of the mechanical events, followed by three curves that represent the pressure changes in the aorta, the left ventricle, and the left atrium. Next is a volume curve that illustrates the changes in volume during the cardiac cycle. The familiar electrocardiographic waveform and a phonocardiogram, or a record of the sounds that are produced by the heart as it pumps, are also included. *A-V,* atrioventricular; *a, c,* and *v,* atrial pressure waves.

*Source:* Reprinted from *Textbook of Medical Physiology* by A.C. Guyton, p. 164, with permission of W.B. Saunders Company, © 1976.

The P wave is generated by the depolarization of the atria. The normal duration of the P wave is approximately 0.10 second. The QRS complex occurs about 0.16 second after the start of the P wave and represents depolarization of the ventricles. It takes approximately 0.08 second ( ± 0.02) to complete the QRS complex. Shortly after, the T wave, or the ventricular repolarization wave, occurs. The T wave marks the beginning of diastole, when the ventricular muscles begin to relax. These electrical events occur shortly before their respective mechanical events (see Figure 1–15). As noted earlier, it is the electrical event that initiates the mechanical event.

*Mechanical Events*

It is possible to divide the mechanical events of the cardiac cycle into seven sequential phases. In order, from beginning diastole to end-systole, the events are

1. isometric relaxation
2. rapid inflow
3. diastasis
4. atrial systole
5. isometric contraction
6. ejection
7. protodiastole

For the purposes of this discussion, the phases will be described only as they occur in the left chambers of the heart; however, the same events occur in the right chambers of the heart.

At the conclusion of ventricular systole, most of the blood that was available for ejection from the left ventricle has been ejected. (See the volume curve in Figure 1–15.) Because of the reduced ventricular volume and the relaxation of the ventricular muscle fibers, the pressure in the ventricle falls. When it falls below the pressure in the aorta, the higher pressure in the aorta pushes blood toward the aortic leaflets, causing them to snap closed. At this point, with the closure of the aortic valves and the occurrence of the second heart sound ($S_2$), which this closure produces, diastole begins. It consists of four of the seven mechanical phases of the cardiac cycle.

The first phase of diastole is isometric or isovolumic relaxation. During this phase, all valves are closed; and the ventricular volume cannot change; however, the muscle fibers continue to relax, causing the intraventricular pressure to fall very rapidly to its low diastolic level. When the left intraventricular pressure is lower than the left intra-atrial pressure, the mitral valve leaflets are pushed open, and ventricular filling begins.

The rapid inflow phase is the second phase of ventricular diastole and the first phase of ventricular filling. It consumes approximately one-third of the ventricular filling time. As stated, this phase begins with the opening of the atrioventricular valve. Blood rapidly passes from the atrium into the ventricle, thus rapidly increasing the volume in the ventricle. The intra-atrial pressure falls very quickly with the opening of the mitral valve, and the pressures of the two chambers become very similar.

The middle third of ventricular filling, or diastasis, is a period of very slow filling. The blood that enters the atrium flows passively into the ventricle, bringing the ventricular volume to approximately 70 percent of its capacity.[29] During this phase, the leaflets of the mitral valve begin to float closed; before they can completely close, however, they are forced open by contraction of the atrial muscles. This valve motion can be seen clearly on an echocardiogram.

Atrial systole completes the filling portion of ventricular diastole. During this phase, the atrial muscles contract, force the mitral leaflets to a fully open position, and contribute the final 30 percent of the total ventricular volume. Under normal circumstances, the heart can perform very adequately without this extra volume, as is often seen clinically in individuals with atrial tachyarrhythmias. In those individuals whose cardiac reserve is depleted, however, the loss of 30 percent of ventricular volume because of the loss of atrial systole, or atrial kick, can be catastrophic.

At the end of diastole, just before the atrioventricular valves snap closed and produce the first heart sound ($S_1$), the intraventricular pressure, the intra-atrial pressure, the pulmonary vein, the pulmonary capillary, and the pulmonary artery pressures are all essentially the same, ranging from 4 to 13 mm Hg. This occurs because the mitral valve is open and the pulmonary vascular system is open back to the closed pulmonic valve. This fact is the reason that left ventricular performance can be evaluated via pulmonary artery pressure monitoring in the clinical setting.

Ventricular systole begins with the contraction of the ventricular muscle fibers. As the fibers contract, the intraventricular pressure rises. When this pressure exceeds the intra-atrial pressure, the mitral valve leaflets are forced to their closed position. The period of isometric or isovolumic contraction has begun. During this very brief phase, 0.02 to 0.03 second, the pressure within the ventricle rises very rapidly, building up the force required to eject the ventricle's contents into the aorta.[30] Again, the volume does not change during this phase, because all valves are closed.

Once the pressure in the ventricle is great enough to overcome the intra-aortic diastolic pressure, the semilunar valve is pushed open. This ends the period of isometric contraction and begins the period of ventricular ejection. Immediately after the opening of the aortic valve, blood begins to flow out of the ventricle. Approximately 60 percent of the ventricular emptying occurs during the first one-fourth of systole; most of the remaining 40 percent occurs during the next two fourths.[31] At this point, ventricular ejection is essentially complete, and the last portion of systole, protodiastole, begins.

Protodiastole consumes the last one-fourth of systole. During this phase, the ventricular muscles remain contracted, but little blood is ejected. Any flow of blood into the aorta at this time is probably the result of momentum that was built up during earlier portions of the ejection phase. With the movement of blood out of the ventricle and then out of the aorta toward the peripheral vasculature, pressures in the ventricle and aorta fall. As the ventricular muscle fibers begin to relax, the intraventricular pressure continues to fall; when it becomes lower than the intra-aortic pressure, the aortic valve snaps closed. This ends the period of systole, and a new cardiac cycle begins.

The increase in systolic intraventricular pressure overcomes the diastolic intra-aortic pressure and opens the aortic valve (see Figure 1–15). For a period of time during systole, then, the two pressures are essentially the same, peaking at approximately 120 mm Hg. When the ventricular pressure falls far enough below the aortic pressure to allow the higher aortic pressure to force the valve leaflets to close, blood is flowing both forward toward the periphery and, to a small extent, back toward the aortic valve. With the closure of the valve, a backflow pressure against the aortic valve increases pressure. This is depicted as an incisura or notch on the aortic waveform. Frequently, the incisura is referred to as the dicrotic notch. After this brief rise, the aortic pressure continues to fall slowly throughout diastole to approximately 80 mm Hg at end-diastole.

Simultaneously with the events of ventricular systole and diastole, pressure events occur within the atria. The a wave is caused by atrial contraction (see Figure 1–15). When the ventricles begin to contract, the atrioventricular valves bulge back because of the rising ventricular pressure and the pull of the contracting ventricular muscles on the atrial muscles. These two factors cause the c atrial wave. The v wave, associated with the end of ventricular contraction, is due to the rise in atrial pressure as blood flows from the pulmonary veins into the left atrium. The v wave disappears after the opening of the atrioventricular valve.

In the clinical setting, it is essential for the practitioner to know the normal pressures in the heart chambers and the pulmonary and aortic vasculature during the cardiac cycle (Table 1–1). It is also important to recognize the similarity of pressures in certain areas during systole or diastole.

**Regulation of Muscle Mechanics**

The purpose of the heart is to pump sufficient oxygenated blood through the circulatory system to meet the metabolic needs of the tissues of the body. Those factors that regulate the muscle mechanics of the heart and, therefore, cardiac performance, are of obvious importance. The regulatory factors can be divided into two categories: intrinsic and extrinsic.

**Table 1–1** Normal Pressures* in the Heart Chambers and Great Arteries

|  | Systolic (mm Hg) | Diastolic (mm Hg) | Mean (mm Hg) |
|---|---|---|---|
| Right atrium | | | −1−+8 |
| Right ventricle | 15–28 | 0–8 | |
| Pulmonary artery | 15–28 | 5–16 | 10–22 |
| Pulmonary capillary | | | 6–15 |
| Left atrium | | | 4–12 |
| Left ventricle | 90–140 | 4–12† | |
| Aorta | 90–140 | 60–90 | 70–105 |

*Measured at one-half of anteroposterior chest diameter in recumbent, normal adults.
†Left ventricular end-diastolic pressure.

*Intrinsic Regulation*

Those contractile properties inherent in the muscle fibers themselves are the intrinsic regulators of cardiac muscle function. Involved are the mechanisms of (1) preload, or the length of the muscle fibers at the onset of contraction; (2) afterload, or the force that the heart must develop to overcome impedance to ventricular ejection; (3) contractility, or the ability of the heart to contract independent of variations in preload or afterload; (4) homeometric autoregulation, or the increase in ventricular performance with no change in muscle fiber length; and (5) heart rate, or frequency of contraction. Although separate, these mechanisms are interrelated.

**Preload.** The basic concept underlying the regulating mechanism of preload is Starling's law of the heart. This law states that the more the heart is filled or stretched during diastole, the greater the force or tension developed by the ventricle for the next contraction (Figure 1–16). The length-tension relationship is the means by which the heart adapts to varying volumes. When the cardiac muscle fibers are stretched because of an increased volume within the chamber at the end of diastole, the greater force of the next contraction automatically pumps the extra volume to the arterial vasculature. Consequently, the heart is able, within physiologic limits, to pump the varying volumes of blood that come to it and prevent a backup in the venous system. This concept is analogous to the stretching of a rubber band. If the rubber band is stretched only a small amount, the force of the next contraction is low; if the rubber band is stretched a great distance, however, the result is a very forceful contraction.

Another term used to describe Starling's law is *heterometric autoregulation*, an inherent, intrinsic property of the muscle fiber that is evident in the heart even in the absence of all neural or humoral influences. It is theorized that this property is

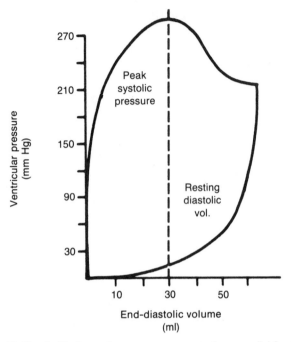

**Figure 1–16** Classic Starling volume-pressure curve of myocardial function. Within physiologic limits, increased end-diastolic ventricular volume results in increased peak ventricular pressure. Beyond the broken line, the ventricle is overstretched, and the heart responds to increased filling with less pressure.

*Sources:* Reprinted from *Journal of Physiology,* Vol. 48, p. 465, with permission of The Physiological Society, © 1914; *Circulatory Physiology* by J.J. Smith and J.P. Kampine, p. 78, with permission of Williams & Wilkins Company, Baltimore, © 1984.

due to the coupling of a greater number of myosin cross-bridges with active sites on the actin filaments. The length of a myocardial fiber at which maximal force develops is approximately 2.2 μm, and it is at this length that the actin and myosin filaments are optimally overlapped to allow the greatest number of cross-bridge interactions.

In the clinical setting, the measure for preload is the pulmonary artery end-diastolic pressure or left atrial pressure. These pressures can be used in most clinical situations, because like the pulmonary capillary pressure, they are very similar to the left ventricular end-diastolic pressure (see Table 1–1). This ventricular pressure is an indicator of left ventricular end-diastolic volume, or the presystolic load that the ventricle must move with the subsequent contraction.

**Afterload.** The total load on the heart includes preload and afterload. Afterload may be defined as the load that the cardiac muscle must move after it begins to contract or as the pressure that the cardiac muscle must develop before its fibers can begin to shorten. If the heart is to eject a volume of blood, it must overcome any impediments to its purpose. The major impeding force for the left ventricle is an aortic pressure that is strong enough to hold the aortic valve leaflets in a closed position, thus preventing the flow of blood from the ventricle to the aorta and peripheral vascular system. The aortic pressure, however, is not the only factor that impedes left ventricular ejection. Other factors include

- the resistance to flow presented by the aortic valve, which is minimal in the normal heart but significant with a stenotic valve
- the distensibility of the vascular system
- peripheral vascular resistance
- reflected pressure waves in the aorta

All these factors act in combination to create the load that the left ventricle must move after it begins to contract. Similar forces in the pulmonary system create the afterload of the right ventricle.

The influence of the afterload on the contracting muscle can be seen in the sequence of changes in tension, or force, and length that the muscle fibers undergo during each cardiac cycle. During diastole, when the fibers are relaxed, the volume of blood in the ventricle stretches the fibers, creating a certain tension and pressure. At the outset of the contractile phase or isovolumic contraction, the muscle fibers attempt to shorten, but cannot do so because not enough tension has built up to overcome the resisting load or afterload (see Figure 1–15). When the tension that builds up during this phase equals the opposing force, the fibers begin to shorten, the semilunar valves open, and blood is ejected—the ventricular ejection phase (see Figure 1–15). Toward the end of systole, the fibers begin to relax; this phase of contraction compares to protodiastole (see Figure 1–15). During this phase, the load (aortic pressure) is returned to its original resting position; thus, the semilunar valves close, freeing the ventricle of its afterload. At this point, isovolumic relaxation begins. Tension within the muscle declines rapidly, because there is essentially no load and certainly no afterload to influence the ventricular myocardium. This phase ends when the pressure falls below that in the atrium and blood fills the ventricle, generating the next preload.

The degree of afterload and the force generated can be related to the rate or velocity of myofibril shortening. The force that the muscle can develop is dependent on the number of cross-bridges that interact at a given time. The velocity with which the muscle fibers shorten depends on the rate at which the cross-bridges can attach, pull, detach, and return to their original configuration. The force-velocity relationship is an inverse one (Figure 1–17). If the afterload is large, the heart contracts slowly; if the afterload is small, the rate of contraction is faster. For

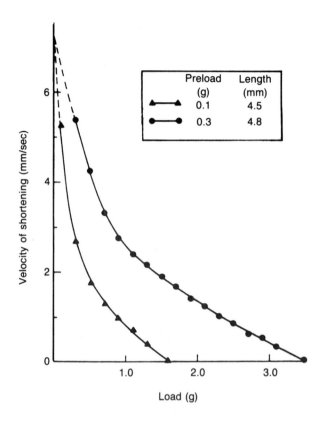

**Figure 1–17** Effect of increasing initial muscle length on force-velocity relationship of a cat papillary muscle. The initial velocity of shortening is plotted against the afterload for each curve. Increasing the initial muscle length increases the maximum force of contraction with no change in the maximum velocity of shortening.

*Source:* Reprinted with permission from *Federation Proceedings,* Vol. 24, p. 1398, © 1965.

example, the average person can lift a 5-pound weight in one hand very quickly, but that person can lift a 100-pound weight only very slowly, even if both hands are used.

Afterload is also related to the extent of shortening, and the extent of shortening influences the volume ejected. If the preload is held constant, an increase in the afterload will decrease muscle shortening. The result is a decrease in the volume ejected by the ventricle.

It is clinically difficult to obtain a true measure of afterload because of the variables involved in producing the load. Consequently, the total peripheral vascular resistance, also known as systemic vascular resistance, or the mean arterial pressure is often used as an index of impedance to ventricular ejection.

**Contractility.** An intrinsic property of the heart that is difficult to define precisely, contractility has been described as the ability of the heart to contract independent of variations in preload or afterload. The physiologic basis for this property is not clearly understood. Experimentally, determination of the maximum velocity of contraction can be used as a measure of contractility. Clinically, however, there is no available measure for this regulating mechanism. Changes in contractility are generally initiated by extrinsic factors.

**Homeometric Autoregulation.** Closely related to contractility is the concept of homeometric autoregulation. This term is currently used to describe any change that occurs in myocardial contractility without a change in muscle length or preload. Originally, the term was used to describe the cardiac response to an abrupt increase in aortic pressure, the response being an initial decrease followed by a temporary increase in stroke work. This intrinsic, inotropic response of the myocardium is also known as the Anrep effect. Present research evidence indicates that this phenomenon, which may improve coronary blood flow, is of minor importance in the intact human heart.

**Heart Rate.** Alteration of the heart rate and the heart rate interval affects the contractile response of the myofibril in several ways. A change in the heart rate alters the preload because of the change in diastolic filling time. In addition, a rate increased into the tachycardiac range has a positive inotropic effect. This force-interval relationship, known as treppe, staircase phenomenon, or Bowditch effect, is evidently related to a slight imbalance between the influx and efflux of cellular calcium.

When the interval between beats is longer than normal, as in a sinus exit block, or when there is a pause after an extrasystole, the contractions associated with the next several beats are stronger than are normal contractions. This produces a reverse staircase effect. In the case of a pause after an extrasystole, however, the premature depolarization itself reduces the inotropic effect. The magnitude of this reduction depends on how early the extrasystole occurs.

*Extrinsic Regulation*

Factors outside the heart that may affect its inotropic or contractile state are described as extrinsic regulatory factors. Generally, there are three types of extrinsic factors: (1) neurohumoral effects, or those influences of the sympathetic or parasympathetic systems or of circulating catecholamines; (2) chemical or pharmacologic effects, or those resulting from changes in blood levels of potassium or calcium, alterations in pH, or drugs (e.g., digitalis, calcium antagonists, or sympathetic blocking agents); and (3) pathological effects, or those secondary to muscle damage from myocardial ischemia or toxic effects of chemicals or bacteria.

Sympathetic stimulation; increased levels of circulating catecholamines; and injection of digitalis, its derivatives, or calcium ions produce positive inotropic effects. Application of any of these stimuli to the intact heart elevates the maximum velocity, shifting the force-velocity curve upward and to the right (Figure 1–18, A). With sympathetic stimulation, the Starling curve is shifted upward and to the left (Figure 1–18, B). Myocardial ischemia, hypocalcemia, hyperkalemia, toxic and anesthetic agents, or cardiac failure creates a negative inotropic effect. This change in the inotropic state is manifested by a lower Starling curve and lower force-velocity curve with a decreased maximum velocity (Figure 1–18).

## Cardiac Output

The volume ejected from the left ventricle to the aorta per minute is the cardiac output. Another term that may be interchanged with cardiac output is minute volume. Cardiac output (CO) is the product of stroke volume (SV), the volume ejected with each ventricular systole or stroke, and the heart rate (HR), which can be expressed as the following equation.

$$CO = SV \times HR$$

The cardiac output for a healthy adult man is approximately 5.6 liters/min; for a woman, it is approximately 4.75 liters/min, or 10 to 20 percent less than that of a

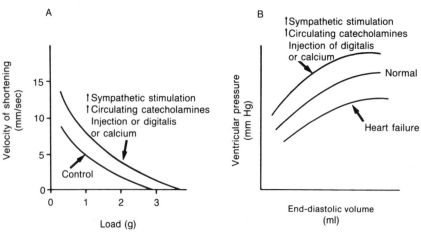

**Figure 1–18** Inotropic effects on the myocardial force-velocity curve (A) and on the ventricular volume-pressure curve (B).

man. The range of values for healthy adults of both sexes and all ages is approximately 4 to 6 liters/min.

It is probably of more clinical value to consider the cardiac output in relation to body size than to consider the absolute value. A tall, heavy individual is likely to require a greater cardiac output than is a short, thin person. In order to compare the cardiac output of individuals, practitioners use the measure of cardiac index (*CI*). The cardiac index is the cardiac output divided by the body surface area (*BSA*) in square meters. This can be expressed by the following formula:

$$CI = CO/BSA$$

The normal cardiac index ranges from 2.8 to 4.2 liters/min/m$^2$.[32]

In an organism of fixed mass, the metabolic rate is the overriding determinant of total flow. Consequently, cardiac output requirements rise appreciably when metabolic demands increase (e.g., because of fever, exercise, or hyperthyroidism) and diminish when metabolic demands decrease (e.g., during sleep or in conditions such as hypothyroidism). These changes in cardiac output are stimulated by the needs of the body, rather than by the heart itself. Therefore, the heart does not regulate its own output, but instead pumps the minimum volume required.

Regulation of the pump function of the heart is a complex interaction of a variety of factors. These factors can be divided into two major categories: systemic factors that affect the return of blood to the heart and cardiac factors that affect the ability of the heart to pump out the blood returned to it.

*Systemic Influences on Cardiac Output*

The primary factor that affects the return of blood to the heart, or venous return, is the force forwarded through the arteries and veins by left ventricular ejection. Sometimes called the systemic filling pressure, this force represents the hemodynamic gradient for all systemic circulation, beginning at the aortic root and ending at the right atrium. This pressure is approximately 7 mm Hg in humans.[33] The difference between the systemic filling pressure and the right atrial pressure (i.e., the force opposing the return of blood) is the net driving pressure that returns blood to the heart. At normal values of 7 mm Hg for the systemic filling pressure and near 0 for the right atrial pressure, the 7-mm gradient produces a venous flow of approximately 5.5 liters/min. Thus, venous flow is essentially the same as cardiac output.

A similar driving force in the pulmonary system affects the flow of blood from the right ventricle to the left atrium. This is the mean pulmonary filling pressure. Normally, it is approximately 2 mm Hg in humans. A number of secondary factors also influence venous return.

**Skeletal Muscle Pump.** When an individual stands, blood moves toward the lower extremities and begins to pool there, thus increasing the hydrostatic pressures of the foot and ankle veins. Shortly after this, the lower extremity skeletal muscles unconsciously begin rhythmic cycles of contraction and relaxation. The muscle contractions squeeze the blood toward the heart; the venous valves prevent the blood from flowing back. During relaxation, the veins refill from below.

The effectiveness of the skeletal muscle pump depends on the competence of the venous valves, the rate of venous inflow in the lower extremities, and the counterweight against which the muscles contract. Venous inflow is related to the temperature of the extremity. If the legs are cool, at 25°C, for example, the inflow is less, and the effectiveness of the skeletal muscle pump is great. If their temperature is 39°C, however, inflow is great, and the skeletal pump is less effective. This explains the intolerance of patients with heart failure for quiet standing in hot weather.

Lack of a counterweight against which the muscles of the extremities can contract when the body is suspended in the upright position also reduces the effectiveness of the skeletal pump. That is, suspending someone in an upright, dangling position for 20 to 40 minutes will result in fainting; a longer suspension can be life-threatening. This occurs because the unconscious rhythmic contraction and relaxation of the skeletal muscles is rendered ineffective without the counterweight of the floor or other surface.

**Venous Valves.** As already mentioned, the venous valves are thin, cusplike structures that promote unidirectional flow. They are located in the veins of the neck and extremities. As discussed previously, competent valves are essential to efficient muscle pump action.

**Venomotor Tone.** The smooth muscles of the venous walls respond to a variety of humoral and neural stimuli. Contraction of these muscles causes venoconstriction during stress, exercise, and marked hypotension in order to increase venous return. Sympathomimetic drugs and cardiac glycosides are also known to produce venoconstriction. Sympatholytic agents and drugs that directly dilate the veins produce venous pooling, thus decreasing venous return.

**Intrathoracic Pressure.** The mean intrathoracic pressure is usually negative, approximately $-2$ to $-4$ mm Hg during expiration and $-5$ to $-7$ mm Hg during inspiration.[34] This negative pressure promotes venous flow into the heart from the systemic vessels. Venous return is increased during inspiration, resulting in an approximately 20-ml increase in the right ventricular stroke volume. Simultaneously, the left ventricular filling and stroke volume are reduced because of the increased capacity of the pulmonary vessels during inspiration. With expiration, this process is reversed so that the left ventricular output varies only about 5 to 7 percent during a full respiratory cycle.[35]

Elevation of the intrathoracic pressure, as with positive pressure respiration or pneumothorax, impedes venous return. This diminishes ventricular filling volume and ultimately reduces ventricular performance.

**Intrapericardial Pressure.** An increase in intrapericardial pressure, as occurs in pericardial effusion, impedes cardiac filling. This reduces the filling and, thus, the performance of the ventricle.

**Ventricular Action on the Atria.** During ventricular contraction, when the atrioventricular valves are closed, the ventricles pull the atrioventricular valve rings downward. This action enlarges the atria and, thus, lowers their internal pressures. Venous flow from the venae cavae and pulmonary veins is increased because of the reduced pressure gradient.

*Cardiac Influences on Cardiac Output*

Because cardiac output is the product of stroke volume and heart rate, alterations in either or both of these parameters change the cardiac output. Such changes may be necessary to maintain the cardiac output at the appropriate level if there are alterations in venous return or metabolic demands.

**Control of Stroke Volume.** The amount of blood ejected by the ventricle with each contraction is the stroke volume. It is not equal to preload, however. The heart does not pump all the blood volume that is available to it, but holds a portion in reserve. The amount left in the ventricle at the end of systole is the end-systolic volume. Stroke volume (*SV*) then is the difference between the end-diastolic volume (*EDV*) and the end-systolic volume (*ESV*):

$$SV = EDV - ESV$$

Stroke volume can be related to end-diastolic volume in an expression termed the ejection fraction. The ejection fraction (*EF*) is calculated by means of the following formula:

$$EF = SV/EDV$$

This calculation is a measure of the pump function of the left ventricle as it is affected by factors that control cardiac output. The normal ejection fraction in humans is 0.50 to 0.75.[36]

The primary determinants of stroke volume are the same primary intrinsic factors that regulate muscle mechanics: preload, contractility, afterload, and heart rate. Consequently, any alteration in one of these regulatory mechanisms alters cardiac output.

Preload is the major factor in maintaining a balance between venous return and stroke volume. If the preload is too low, the stroke volume decreases. If the venous return is increased for any reason, the cardiac muscle is able to accommodate the additional load by contracting with a greater force, although there are physiologic limits to this regulating mechanism. Optimal stretch is 2.2 μm, but this is not a clinically useful measure; an optimal pulmonary artery end-diastolic pressure is used. The optimal pulmonary artery end-diastolic pressure for patients suffering from an acute myocardial infarction, for example, has been identified as 20 to 24 mm Hg, with normal being less than 12 mm Hg.[37]

As indicated earlier, the inotropic state of the cardiac myofibrils allows the heart to contract with more strength and velocity at a constant preload and/or afterload. The result is a more complete emptying of the ventricle, or a reduced end-systolic volume with an increased stroke volume. This causes higher systolic pressures in both the ventricle and the aorta.

Changes in aortic pressure, or afterload, result in inverse changes in the strength, velocity, and duration of left ventricular ejection and, consequently, stroke volume. At normal pressures (i.e., mean arterial pressure of 70 to 105 mm Hg or systemic vascular resistance of 900 to 1,400 dynes-sec/cm$^{-5}$), however, cardiac output is relatively independent of afterload. If the stroke volume is briefly reduced by a moderate rise in arterial pressure, the pumping action of the right ventricle maintains the left ventricular filling pressure and end-diastolic volume. Together with homeometric autoregulation, this action restores the stroke volume.

An increase in the heart rate shortens the ventricular filling time in diastole. This reduces ventricular filling pressure and volume, thus reducing stroke volume as well. The increased heart rate first encroaches on the slow filling phase or diastasis, however, and ventricular filling occurs primarily during the rapid filling phase; therefore, a moderate rise in heart rate has a minimal effect on diastolic filling. Heart rates up to 180 beats/min secondary to sympathetic stimulation or exercise provide an adequate stroke volume in young adults if atrial filling pressures are maintained. This is because of the combined effects of increased venous return with increased atrial pressure, increased strength of ventricular contractions, and a shortening of ventricular systole with a relative lengthening of diastole. If heart rates are artificially increased secondary to a mechanical pacemaker, however, cardiac output first rises, then levels off, and finally begins to decline at rates of 120 to 130 beats/min. This occurs because other regulating mechanisms, such as increased inotropy, have not been activated.

**Control of Heart Rate.** In addition to its direct influence on stroke volume, the heart rate affects cardiac output independent of stroke volume. If the stroke volume were held constant, an increase in the heart rate would increase the cardiac output; conversely, if the heart rate were held constant, an increase in stroke volume would increase the cardiac output. The key factor in the heart rate is the rate of impulse formation in the sinoatrial node. This impulse formation is determined primarily by (1) the autonomic balance between the sympathetic and parasympathetic influences on the node, (2) temperature and metabolic activity of the pacemaker tissue, and (3) less importantly, the effect of ionic and pH changes on the heart.

Both sympathetic and parasympathetic nerve fibers richly innervate the heart. Sympathetic fibers are distributed to the sinoatrial node, atrioventricular node, muscle of the atria, and muscle of the ventricles. Parasympathetic fibers, on the other hand, are distributed mainly to the sinoatrial node, atrioventricular node, and, to a lesser extent, the atrial muscle. These two components of the autonomic nervous system affect cardiac performance by changing the heart rate and the strength with which the heart muscle fibers contract. The sympathetic system increases the heart rate and the force of contraction; the parasympathetic system decreases the heart rate and contractility.

Stimulation of the sympathetic nervous system increases the rate of sinoatrial node discharge, which enhances the rate of conduction and the excitability of all portions of the heart. Contractility of both atrial and ventricular muscle fibers is increased by as much as 100 percent with maximal stimulation. When the sympathetic system is stimulated, the nerve endings release norepinephrine. It is believed that this hormone increases the permeability of the cell membrane to sodium and calcium. Such an increased permeability to sodium causes the resting potential of the sinoatrial node to rise to the threshold level more quickly, increasing the rate of self-excitation (Figure 1–19). Increased sodium permeability in the atrioventricular node makes it easier for each cell to excite the

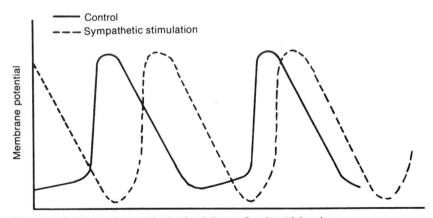

Figure 1–19 Effects of sympathetic stimulation on the sinoatrial node.

next, decreasing the conduction time from the upper chambers to the ventricles. The increased permeability of cells to calcium enhances contractility.[38]

The effect of parasympathetic stimulation on the heart is to decrease both the rate at which impulses are discharged from the sinoatrial node and the rate at which atrial impulses are transmitted to the ventricles; the latter results from the decrease in excitability of the atrioventricular nodal cells. These two parasympathetic effects are caused by the release of acetylcholine from the parasympathetic nerve endings, which increases the permeability of the cell membrane to potassium. The increased permeability allows the potassium ion to leak rapidly from the cell, producing a greater negativity inside the cell, hyperpolarization. This makes it more difficult to excite the cell (Figure 1–20).[39] In addition to the parasympathetic effect on impulse discharge and conduction, stimulation of the parasympathetic system decreases ventricular contractile strength, but only by approximately 30 percent with maximal stimulation.[40]

Clearly, the sympathetic and parasympathetic systems have opposing effects on the heart rate. The cardioinhibitory effects of the parasympathetic system mediate the cardiostimulatory effects of the sympathetic system. Consequently, a balance between the two is necessary if the heart rate is to remain within a normal range. Stimulation of either component of the autonomic nervous system alters the heart rate.

Mechanoreceptors in the wall of the right atrium at the venocaval junction shift the autonomic balance in favor of the sympathetic system. When the receptors are stretched, either by the administration of large volumes of intravenous solutions or by the accumulation of blood, they transmit afferent signals through the vagus nerve to the medulla of the brain. Efferent signals are sent back through the sympathetic nerves to the sinoatrial node, causing it to generate impulses more rapidly. Interestingly, the contractile response to sympathetic stimulation is not affected.[41] This reflex tachycardia, known as the Bainbridge reflex, depends on

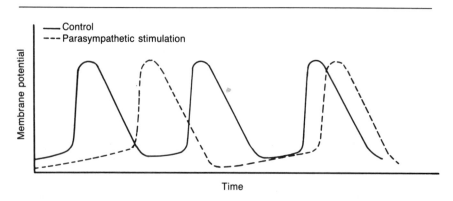

Figure 1–20 Effects of parasympathetic stimulation on the sinoatrial node.

the heart rate at the time of the volume load. If the rate is less than 110 beats/min, the heart rate increases, with an increase in venous return. On the other hand, if the rate is greater than 110 beats/min, the response is cardiac slowing.[42]

The heart rate increases when the body temperature or metabolic rate increases, and decreases when they decrease. The heart rate change secondary to body temperature changes is likely the result of the influence of temperature on the permeability of the cell membrane to ions. The change in permeability alters the self-excitation or spontaneous depolarization in phase 4 of the sinoatrial node action potential. A temperature change of 1°C results in a rate change of approximately 10 beats/min.

Alterations in ionic concentrations can affect the heart rate by means of the changes that they elicit in the action potentials of pacemaker and conductive cells. It is particularly important to monitor potassium ion concentrations because of their influence on the excitability of the cardiac cells. Increased extracellular potassium decreases the excitability of these cells by hyperpolarizing them, resulting in a slowing of the heart rate (see Figure 1–20). In addition, hyperkalemia reduces the rate of increase and amplitude of the action potential, slows the conduction velocity, and accelerates repolarization, thus shortening the plateau phase (i.e., phase 2).

A functional change in any of the mechanisms influences the function of others to some extent. The mechanism that plays the dominant role in controlling cardiac output at any given time depends on the existing stroke volume and heart rate at that time. Studies show, however, that heart rate is more important than stroke volume in making major temporary adjustments in cardiac output.[43]

## Cardiac Energetics

The energy source for cardiac contraction, ATP, is obtained from the metabolism of a variety of substrates, including glucose, fatty acids, lactate, ketone bodies, and amino acids. This metabolic energy is converted into pressure and tension in a series of steps that includes

- conversion of substrate energy into myocardial wall tension
- transference of wall tension into intracardiac pressure
- utilization of these forces, pressure and tension, to eject blood[44]

The type of load, the geometry of the ventricles, the level of contractility, and the heart rate influence the amount of energy that the heart consumes and the efficiency with which it converts the energy to useful work.

*Cardiac Metabolism*

The heart can produce ATP by the metabolic pathways of glycolysis and oxidative phosphorylation. The major energy-generating reaction in the heart is oxidative phosphorylation, but glycolytic reactions are essential for aerobic breakdown of carbohydrate and for ATP production in anaerobic conditions.

Under normal conditions, the heart uses the substrate that is present in the largest concentration. After a meal of carbohydrate, for example, the concentration of glucose is higher, and glucose becomes the primary energy source. If the arterial concentration of glucose is above 60 mg/dl, insulin, epinephrine, anoxia, and increased cardiac work facilitate the diffusion of glucose into the myocardial cell. Inside the cell, glucose undergoes phosphorylation to glucose-6-phosphate (G-6-P) and either is converted to glycogen or enters the glycolytic energy pathway via conversion to fructose-6-phosphate (Figure 1–21). Further conversion to fructose-1,6-diphosphate leads to the production of pyruvic acid.

With normal oxygen availability, the pyruvate is converted to acetyl-coenzyme A (CoA) and enters the citric acid or Krebs' cycle in the mitochondria. Via oxidative phosphorylation, it is converted into high-energy bonds of ATP. In this full oxidative reaction, 36 ATP molecules are produced. In the anaerobic state, however, pyruvate does not enter the citric acid cycle, but is converted to lactic acid. In this event, only 2 ATP molecules are produced.

In the postabsorptive state, the heart shifts to metabolism of fatty acids and ketones. Fatty acids are normally the major energy source. They passively enter the myocardium as long as their blood concentration is above a threshold level of approximately 0.35 mmol. Once inside the cell, the fatty acids are bound to intracellular proteins; after activation to free fatty acids, however, they can be converted to tissue lipids or enter the citric acid cycle in the mitochondria in the form of acetyl-CoA. Beyond the citric acid cycle, phosphorylation occurs, producing ATP (see Figure 1–21).

As can be seen from the preceding discussion, the heart is dependent on an adequate supply of substrate and oxygen. Oxygen is essential for the production of 95 percent of the ATP during carbohydrate metabolism and 100 percent of the ATP during fatty acid metabolism. Consequently, in the anaerobic state, only 5 to 7 percent of the normal energy production is possible. Without adequate energy, cardiac function rapidly deteriorates.

*Myocardial Wall Tension*

The relationship between myocardial wall tension and ventricular pressure or volume can be demonstrated by the law of LaPlace if it is assumed that the left ventricle is spheroid and that the myocardial fibers are oriented in the same

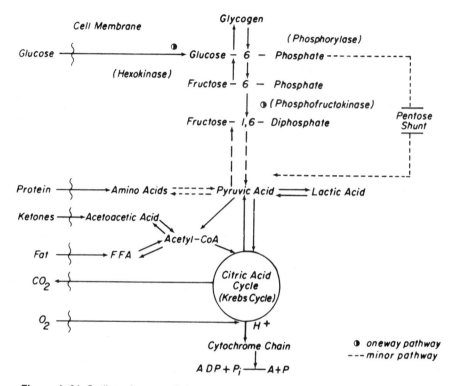

**Figure 1–21** Outline of myocardial metabolism, showing the major steps and principal enzymes in the glycolytic pathways. *FFA,* free fatty acids.

*Source:* Reproduced with permission from R.C. Little: *Physiology of the Heart & Circulation,* 3rd ed., p. 184. Copyright © 1985 by Year Book Medical Publishers, Inc., Chicago.

direction around the sphere's circumference. In its simplest form and expressed for a thin-walled sphere, the law is

$$T = P \times R$$

where $T$ is wall tension (dynes per centimeter), $P$ is pressure (dynes per square centimeter), and $R$ is radius (centimeters). Thus, the law states that wall tension at any given pressure increases as the radius of the chamber, or ventricular volume, increases—and vice versa.

The efficiency with which contractile tension is converted into ventricular pressure is dependent on the size of the heart. This can be seen more clearly if the formula is rearranged as

$$P = T/R$$

In the dilated heart, the wall tension must be greater to produce the same ventricular pressure. Tension can be decreased, however, by increasing the thickness of the wall, thus distributing the tension over a greater number of fibers. This relationship can be written as

$$T = \frac{P \times R}{h}$$

where $h$ is wall thickness.

Because the geometry of the heart and its design do not strictly follow the assumptions made earlier, the calculation of myocardial wall tension is much more complex than is that described by the preceding formulas. The relationships do demonstrate two fundamental facts, however. First, dilation of the ventricles increases tension on each ventricular muscle fiber. Second, an increase in wall thickness decreases the tension on any given muscle fiber. Both of these consequences are of great importance.

*Cardiac Work*

The myocardial transfer of energy from its metabolic substrate to the pressure and kinetic energy of the blood in the vascular system involves two types of cardiac work—external and internal. External work is the energy used in the ejection of the blood against the aortic and pulmonary pressures. Internal work is the energy wasted in the form of heat or used to carry out the normal tissue activities, as well as to open and close the valve cusps. Total cardiac work encompasses both external and internal work and correlates with the oxygen requirements of the heart. It is inferred from the metabolic oxygen demands.

**External Work.** The external cardiac work required depends on the amount of pressure-volume work (i.e., work to eject a given volume at a given pressure) that must be performed and kinetic energy that must be generated. The stroke work (*SW*) is the stroke volume (*SV*) times the pressure (*P*) at which the volume is ejected:

$$SW = SV \times P$$

The amount of external work per minute (*MW*) is calculated by multiplying the stroke work by the heart rate (*HR*):

$$MW = SW \times HR$$

This external or pressure-volume work may also be approximated from the multiplication of the cardiac output (*CO*) and the mean arterial pressure (*MAP*):

$$SW = CO \times MAP$$

Any change, then, in the heart rate, stroke volume, or afterload affects the minute work and the metabolic requirements of the myocardium.

Both ventricles eject the same volume of blood, and both contract at the same rate. Because the mean arterial pressure of the aorta is five to six times that of the pulmonary artery, however, the minute work of the right ventricle is approximately one-sixth that of the left ventricle.

In addition to stroke work, both ventricles perform work to generate the kinetic energy necessary to accelerate the flow of blood. At rest, only about 2 to 4 percent of the useful work of the heart is in the form of kinetic energy. During exercise, however, this fraction may increase to 20 or 25 percent of the total work of the heart.

**Internal Work.** The heart expends a significant amount of energy in the performance of internal work during the cardiac cycle. This includes the expenditure of energy to satisfy the basal metabolic needs of the heart, as well as that to change the shape and length of the contractile components of the wall. This work is wasted in heat and is not quantified.

*Myocardial Oxygen Consumption*

Energy for cardiac work in the normal heart is derived from the oxidative metabolism of substrates. Because the heart can store only minimal amounts of energy in the form of ATP, it must be continuously supplied with oxygen and substrates. Therefore, the amount of energy expended by the heart in its work can be approximated by the amount of oxygen that it uses. Myocardial oxygen consumption is expressed in milliliters of oxygen per minute per 100 g left ventricle. Approximately 20 percent of the oxygen consumed is for basic maintenance; the other 80 percent is for the work of contraction. The normal heart consumes 8 to 15 ml oxygen per minute per 100 g ventricle. The major determinants of myocardial oxygen consumption are ventricular wall tension, heart rate, and velocity of myocardial shortening.

*Cardiac Efficiency*

The ratio of the useful work produced, or external work, to the energy equivalent of oxygen consumption indicates cardiac efficiency:

$$\text{Cardiac efficiency} = \frac{\text{Work}}{\text{Energy equivalent of oxygen consumption}}$$

When calculated in this way, the efficiency of the myocardium has been found to range between 5 and 20 percent, the specific value depending on the amount and nature of the work performed.[45]

Cardiac efficiency increases during volume loading and decreases during pressure loading. Conditions that increase the ventricular volume (e.g., exercise and aortic insufficiency) result in a more energy-efficient heart because the heart expends relatively less energy in ejecting blood (flow work) than in developing pressure (pressure work). In conditions that increase afterload (e.g., systemic arterial hypertension and aortic stenosis), the heart expends a great deal of energy to develop and maintain a pressure sufficient to open the aortic valve, and additional energy is required to eject blood. Consequently, these hearts are less efficient in terms of energy consumption.

With a modest increase in heart rate and a corresponding increase in cardiac output, there is a reduction in cardiac efficiency. More metabolic energy is required for the greater contractility associated with the faster rate, and the internal work associated with the greater number of contractions per unit of time is increased. Clearly, the decreased efficiency of the failing heart deteriorates even further when the tachycardia often associated with heart failure develops.

## Oxygen Transport

The movement of oxygen from the blood in the left heart to the site of its intracellular use is a function of cardiac output, hemoglobin concentration, and hemoglobin oxygen affinity.

### Effect of Cardiac Output on Oxygen Transport

Tissue cells require a given amount of oxygen ($O_2$) per unit of time. The volume of blood from which the oxygen comes is of minimal importance. If the oxygen consumption per unit of time remains constant, the volume of blood from which the required oxygen is extracted depends on the blood flow per unit of time. If the cardiac output is increased, the amount of oxygen extracted from a given amount of blood is reduced, and the venous oxygen content is higher. Conversely, if the cardiac output is reduced, the amount of oxygen extracted from the given amount of blood is increased, and the venous oxygen content is reduced. Thus, cardiac output influences not only oxygen availability, but also venous oxygen content.[46]

### Hemoglobin Concentration

Hemoglobin (Hb) is normally present in a concentration of 12 to 15 g/dl blood. When oxygen enters the bloodstream, most of the oxygen attaches immediately to hemoglobin to form oxyhemoglobin ($HbO_2$). The rest is carried as dissolved oxygen. Hemoglobin has an enormous oxygen capacity; when totally saturated, 1 g hemoglobin holds 1.34 ml oxygen. The oxygen content of blood is the sum of the oxygen attached to hemoglobin and that dissolved in plasma. At the normal arterial partial pressure of oxygen ($Po_2$ of 95 mm Hg), the oxygen content is 19.7 ml oxygen per 100 ml blood, of which 0.03 ml is dissolved in the plasma and 19.4 ml is combined with hemoglobin.

Oxygen saturation reflects the relationship between the amount of oxygen actually combined with hemoglobin and the amount of oxygen with which the hemoglobin is capable of combining. In other words, the oxygen saturation ($So_2$) equals the ratio of oxygen content to capacity minus the dissolved oxygen times 100:

$$So_2 = 100 \times \frac{O_2 \text{ content } - \text{ Dissolved } O_2}{O_2 \text{ capacity } - \text{ Dissolved } O_2}$$

Normally, the saturation of arterial blood is 97 percent; that of venous blood, 75 percent.

The oxygen saturation of hemoglobin is a function of oxygen tension or the partial pressure of oxygen. Thus, various pressures of oxygen produce various degrees of saturation. Plotting the oxygen saturation for various partial pressures of oxygen gives an S-shaped curve known as the hemoglobin dissociation curve (Figure 1–22).

*Hemoglobin Oxygen Affinity*

Because hemoglobin has a strong affinity for oxygen, poorly oxygenated blood readily accepts oxygen in the pulmonary capillary network. This strong affinity for oxygen makes the hemoglobin less willing to give up oxygen to the tissues, however. A number of factors in the blood alter the oxygen affinity:

• hydrogen ion concentration (pH)
• carbon dioxide tension ($Pco_2$)
• temperature
• level of 2,3-diphosphoglycerate (2,3-DPG), a byproduct of glucose metabolism

By altering the hemoglobin oxygen affinity, these factors alter the normal relationships between hemoglobin saturation and oxygen tension. This changes the position of the hemoglobin dissociation curve, or "shifts the curve" (Figure 1–23).

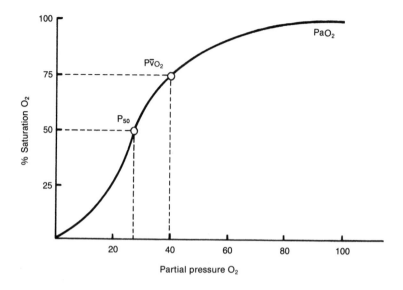

**Figure 1–22** Hemoglobin dissociation curve, showing the relationship between plasma oxygen partial pressure and the degree to which potential oxygen-carrying hemoglobin sites have oxygen attached (% saturation oxygen). Normally, hemoglobin is 50 percent saturated at a plasma $Po_2$ of approximately 27 mm Hg ($P_{50}$). Normal venous blood has an oxygen partial pressure ($Pvo_2$) of 40 mm Hg and an oxyhemoglobin saturation of 75 percent. Normal arterial blood has an oxygen partial pressure ($Pao_2$) of 97 mm Hg and an oxyhemoglobin saturation of 97 percent.

*Source:* Reproduced with permission from B.A. Shapiro, R.A. Harrison, and J.R. Walton: *Clinical Application of Blood Gases,* 3rd ed., p. 81. Copyright © 1982 by Year Book Medical Publishers, Inc., Chicago.

If the hemoglobin dissociation curve shifts to the left, hemoglobin has an increased affinity for oxygen. Therefore, for any given oxygen tension, oxygen saturation is increased. The effect of this increased affinity may be significant with regard to tissue oxygenation, because the transfer of oxygen to the tissue is less effective. Factors that shift the curve to the left are alkalemia (↑pH), hypocapnia (↓$Pco_2$), hypothermia, and decreased levels of 2,3-diphosphoglycerate (↓2,3-DPG).

A shift of the hemoglobin dissociation curve to the right indicates that hemoglobin has a decreased affinity for oxygen. Thus, for any given oxygen tension, oxygen saturation is decreased. Because oxygen content is reduced, the oxygen transport capability of the blood is decreased. Although the hemoglobin gives up its oxygen to the tissues more easily, the reduction in oxygen content limits the amount of oxygen available to the tissues. Factors that decrease hemoglobin's affinity for oxygen are acidemia (↓pH), hypercapnia (↑$Pco_2$), hyperthermia, and increased levels of 2,3-diphosphoglycerate (↑2,3-DPG).

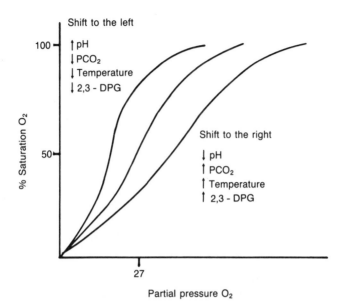

**Figure 1–23** Effects of pH, $P_{CO_2}$, temperature, and 2,3-diphosphoglycerate (2,3-DPG) on the hemoglobin dissociation curve.

Two other factors affect the oxygen saturation–oxygen tension relationship. The first is the hemoglobin itself. If the concentration of hemoglobin is reduced, as it is in anemia, the oxygen capacity and content of blood are reduced. The hemoglobin dissociation curve shifts to the right, because—obviously—less available hemoglobin means less available oxygen. Conversely, polycythemia increases the amount of hemoglobin available and shifts the curve to the left.

The second factor that must also be considered is the affinity of carbon monoxide for hemoglobin. Carbon monoxide binds to hemoglobin, forming carboxyhemoglobin (HbCO), approximately 210 times more easily than does oxygen. Both oxyhemoglobin and carboxyhemoglobin can be present in the blood. In cigarette smokers, for example, as much as 12 percent of their hemoglobin may be bonded to carbon monoxide. This hemoglobin is ineffective in oxygen transport and delivery.[47] High levels of carboxyhemoglobin cause the hemoglobin dissociation curve to shift markedly to the left, because exposure of the blood to carbon monoxide decreases hemoglobin's affinity for oxygen.

**Vascular Performance**

The contribution of the vascular system to cardiac function cannot be overstated.

*Resistance Vessels*

The arterioles offer the major resistance to blood flow. Their smooth muscle layers can vary their wall tension, their diameter, and, therefore, the resistance offered. The totality of the individual resistances, which are inversely proportional to the diameter of the arterioles involved, comprise the systemic vascular resistance. Cardiac output and systemic vascular resistance determine blood pressure, which in turn influences perfusion of tissues. Changes in resistance allow perfusion of individual vascular beds according to their metabolic needs and play a primary role in the regulation of the systemic arterial blood pressure.

**Poiseuille's Law.** Poiseuille, a French physician, described the factors that influence nonpulsatile flow of a homogeneous fluid through rigid tubes. He noted that, if all other factors are held constant, the rate of flow ($Q$) through a length of cylindrical tube ($L$) with a radius ($r$) is directly proportional to the driving pressure ($\Delta P$, the difference in pressure between two ends of the tube). He also noted that flow is inversely proportional to the length of the tube ($L$) and the viscosity of the flowing liquid ($\eta$), but directly proportional to the fourth power of the radius of the tube ($r$). By adding two proportionality constants ($\pi$ and 8), he developed Poiseuille's Law:

$$Q = \Delta P r^4 \pi / \eta L 8$$

Even though blood is a nonhomogeneous fluid that flows through branching distensible tubes in a pulsatile fashion, Poiseuille's law provides helpful approximations in the clinical setting.

**Resistance to Flow.** Factors that may be considered a hindrance to flow are radius to the fourth power, viscosity, and length. If these factors are combined and inverted from their relationship in Poiseuille's law ($\eta L / r^4$) and designated as resistance to flow ($R$), Poiseuille's formula can be simplified to

$$Q = \Delta P / R$$

or transposed to

$$R = \Delta P / Q$$

It is clear that resistance depends on the viscosity of blood, the length of the vessel, and the vessel radius to the fourth power. Because the viscosity of blood and the length of the vessels do not change appreciably over a short period of time, vessel diameter is the most important factor to affect resistance. Vasoconstriction increases the vascular resistance to flow; vasodilation decreases it. Large changes in resistance to flow can be obtained quickly by means of small changes in vessel diameter.

**Regulation of Flow.** The simplified formula $Q = \Delta P/R$ shows that blood flow can be altered either by changing the arterial perfusion pressure or by changing the vessel diameter or resistance. Because it is essential to ensure adequate coronary and cerebral flow, it is best to maintain arterial perfusion pressure at relatively constant levels and to meet peripheral demands for flow by adjusting individual resistances. This can be accomplished either through central regulation or through local regulation of vessel caliber.

Central mechanisms for regulation of flow are those that originate at a site remote from the tissue affected. These mechanisms include both neural and humoral control factors. Neural control of flow is almost exclusively through the autonomic nervous system, which is divided into the sympathetic system and the parasympathetic system. Acetylcholine and norepinephrine are the two primary neurotransmitters of the autonomic nervous system. Acetylcholine is released at all autonomic ganglia, at parasympathetic nerve endings, at voluntary neuromuscular junctions, and at the sympathetic cholinergic endings. Norepinephrine is released at most sympathetic nerve endings.

These neurotransmitters may interact with at least three different receptors at the various anatomical sites. Each receptor responds differently to the neurotransmitters (Table 1–2). When α-receptors, which are abundant in the blood vessels of skin, kidney, splanchnic area, and skeletal muscle, are exposed to norepinephrine or other catecholamines, they produce a strong vasoconstriction. β-Receptors are most prominent in the heart, the blood vessels of skeletal muscles, and the bronchiolar smooth muscles. When activated by the neurotransmitter, they increase the heart rate and contractile strength of the myocardium ($\beta_1$-response) and dilate skeletal muscle blood vessels ($\beta_2$-response). Dopaminergic receptors are located in renal, coronary, splanchnic, and intracerebral vascular beds and produce a vasodilator effect when exposed to low doses of dopamine.

**Table 1–2** Actions of Catecholamines on the Cardiovascular System

| Receptor | Site of Action | Mode of Action |
|---|---|---|
| α | Peripheral vessels | Vasoconstriction |
| $\beta_1$ | Myocardium | Increase in contractility |
|  | Sinus node | Increase in heart rate |
| $\beta_2$ | Peripheral vessels | Vasodilation |
| Dopaminergic | Renal, coronary, splanchnic, and intracerebral arteries | Vasodilation* |

*Response is dose-dependent. With higher doses, the response is vasoconstriction.

Vasoconstriction is accomplished almost entirely by stimulation of the α-receptors. This stimulation increases vascular resistance; increases the central arterial pressure and decreases flow to the constricted vascular beds; reduces capillary hydrostatic pressure, with a resultant net increase in plasma volume; and decreases the caliber of the capacitance vessels, increasing venous return. Vessels can be dilated by one or more of the following four modes:

1. inhibition of the vasoconstrictor center of the medulla
2. stimulation of the sympathetic cholinergic receptors
3. stimulation of the β-sympathetic receptors
4. activation of parasympathetic vasodilators

Humoral control of flow is primarily through circulating catecholamines. Endogenous circulating catecholamines are normally derived from the adrenal medulla, or they may have been released in excessive amounts at the nerve endings. Exogenous circulating catecholamines are those administered intravenously. Whether endogenous or exogenous, the cardiovascular effects are similar to those produced by the sympathetic nervous system. Other humoral vasoactive substances are angiotensin II, vasopressin, serotonin, and several prostaglandins. For the most part, the exact physiologic role of these substances in normal cardiovascular regulation is not yet clear.[48]

Local regulation of blood flow is the result of active hyperemia, reactive hyperemia, or autoregulation. Active hyperemia refers to vasodilation in response to increased metabolism or temperature of the tissues. Accumulated metabolites (e.g., carbon dioxide, lactic acid, potassium ion, and hydrogen ion), as well as decreased $Po_2$ and increased osmolality have been proposed as vasodilator agents. Reactive hyperemia refers to the excessive flow to a tissue when the flow to that tissue has been released after an occlusion. The degree and duration of this afterflow is proportional to the duration of the occlusion. It is thought that the increased flow is due to decreased $Po_2$ or increased metabolites in the tissues. Autoregulation is the intrinsic ability of tissues to keep the local blood flow relatively constant in the face of a changing perfusion pressure. This ability to maintain a consistent flow is particularly advantageous to vital organs, such as the brain and heart.

**Regulation of Blood Pressure**

Blood pressure can be regulated by adjusting the variables of cardiac output and systemic vascular resistance. Both short-term (over minutes and hours) and long-term (over weeks and months) adjustments can be made. The cardiovascular centers of the medulla regulate the blood pressure; however, these centers are governed by higher nervous system centers and many sensors throughout the body. Because some sensors are in the vascular system, the arterial pressure is both the controlled and controlling variable.

**Cardiovascular Centers.** The primary nervous control of circulation lies with the cardiovascular centers in the dorsal reticular matter of the medulla and lower pons. The "centers" are functionally diverse areas that can be divided into the cardiac control area and the vasomotor control area. The former is concerned with neural control of the heart; the latter, with neural control of the peripheral blood vessels. These two divisions are not well defined, resulting in both anatomical and functional overlap between them.

Within the cardiac control area is a distinct cardioinhibitory center. Vagal efferent nerve fibers from these sites transport impulses that slow the heart rate and decrease the contractility of the atria. A cardiostimulatory center has been reported, but its identity as a distinct center is not certain.

A vasoconstrictor center is the major component of the vasomotor control area. The preganglionic fibers of the neurons that descend from this center are primarily responsible for widespread sympathetic vasoconstriction. A distinct vasodilator center is questionable. It is more likely that vasodilation is primarily the result of inhibition of the vasoconstrictor center.

**Intrinsic Reflexes of the Cardiovascular System.** Sensors within the vascular system stimulate intrinsic reflexes. Unlike the extrinsic reflexes (i.e., those that originate in other systems or organs), the intrinsic reflexes are extremely important in the short-term regulation of blood pressure. They are activated by special receptors that are sensitive either to pressure (stretch receptors, baroreceptors, or mechanoreceptors) or to special chemical stimuli (chemoreceptors). Baroreceptors are similar in characteristics, effects, and general functions to cardiopulmonary receptors. Chemoreceptors play a larger role in control of the respiratory system than in control of circulation.

Both baroreceptors and chemoreceptors are located in the walls of the aortic arch and internal carotid arteries. Afferent nerve fibers from these receptors travel via the aortic and carotid sinus nerves, join the vagus or glossopharyngeal nerves, and connect with the cardiovascular centers of the medulla. When the baroreceptor nerve endings are stretched, signals are sent to the vasomotor areas of the medulla, triggering a depressor response and inhibiting a pressor response. Consequently, an elevation of blood pressure produces a reflex action designed to decrease the pressure. In addition, the heart rate and myocardial contractility are reduced. Conversely, if the baroreceptors are understretched because of low blood pressure, a reflex pressor response is stimulated and the depressor response inhibited, resulting in a rise in the blood pressure. In this case, the heart rate and contractility are increased in an attempt to maintain a higher arterial pressure.

Intrathoracic sensors, known as cardiopulmonary receptors, are located at low-pressure sites in the walls of the heart, great vessels, and lungs. These receptors may be found in the atria and the vena cava area, the ventricles, or the pulmonary vascular system. Primarily through the vagal afferent fibers and secondarily through the sympathetic afferent fibers, these receptors activate the medullary cardiovascular centers. The full role of these reflexes in humans is still not known, but animal studies are providing some understanding of their function.

Arterial chemoreceptors are located in the carotid and aortic bodies near the carotid sinus and aortic arch receptors. These special nerve endings respond to a decrease in arterial $Po_2$, an increase in $Pco_2$, or an increase in arterial hydrogen ion concentration. The responses elicited are hyperventilation, sympathetic vasoconstriction, and bradycardia. It seems that the purpose of these receptors is to increase the delivery of oxygen to the brain and heart.

**Extrinsic Reflexes of the Cardiovascular System.** Several stimuli that originate outside the circulatory system are capable of causing cardiovascular responses via afferent nerves. The responses are usually less consistent than those of intrinsic reflexes. For example, the hemodynamic response to pain is variable. Mild to moderate pain usually evokes tachycardia and an increased arterial pressure. Severe pain, however, may bring about bradycardia, hypotension, and perhaps circulatory collapse and fainting. Overly rapid emptying of a hollow organ, as in catheterization of the urinary bladder, may also cause reflex hypotension and, at times, circulatory collapse.

Exposure to local cold may induce vasoconstriction, resulting in an increase in arterial pressure. If the cold temperature is intense, the pressure elevation may be simultaneously stimulated by pain sensors. Patients with coronary artery disease may develop angina secondary to exposure to intense cold because of increased coronary artery resistance and decreased coronary blood flow or because of myocardial ischemia owing to an increased afterload.

**Long-Term Arterial Pressure Regulation.** Long-term control of blood pressure is based on the balance between blood volume and urinary output. This balance is influenced by the renin-angiotensin-aldosterone system. A rise in arterial pressure causes an increased renal output of water and electrolytes; a decreased extracellular fluid volume, blood volume, and venous return; and, consequently, a reduced cardiac output; the low cardiac output prompts a reduction in arterial pressure. Conversely, a decrease in arterial pressure results in retention of fluids and electrolytes by the renal system; increased fluid volume, blood volume, and venous return; and both an increased cardiac output and an increased arterial pressure. At first, the pressure elevation is generally due to the direct effect of an increased cardiac output on the pressure; after several weeks, however, the pressure elevation is primarily due to the indirect effect of the increased peripheral vascular resistance caused by the local autoregulation to increased flow.

*Exchange Vessels*

At the capillary level, the cardiovascular system achieves its true goal. Oxygen and other essential substances are given up to the tissue cells, and carbon dioxide and other metabolites are taken away. This process is accomplished by the combination of diffusion and fluid movement.

**Diffusion.** The exchange of oxygen, carbon dioxide, and other solutes at the capillary level is the result of diffusion along concentration gradients. Lipid-soluble molecules, such as oxygen and carbon dioxide, move across the capillary membrane freely and rapidly. Lipid-insoluble molecules are not free to diffuse across the capillary membrane, however, but are restricted to pores. Small lipid-insoluble molecules, such as water, sodium chloride, urea, and glucose, meet with little resistance to diffusion and, therefore, move rapidly across the membrane, creating an extremely small concentration gradient. Increasingly larger lipid-insoluble molecules meet with increasingly greater resistance, until diffusion becomes minimal with molecules of a molecular weight greater than 60,000.

**Fluid Movement.** The direction and amount of fluid movement across the capillary membrane are determined by the algebraic sum of the hydrostatic and osmotic pressures across the membrane. A high hydrostatic pressure on one side of the membrane favors movement of fluid to the other side, where the hydrostatic pressure is lower. If the osmotic pressure is greater on one side of the capillary membrane because of an increased concentration of osmotically active particles, however, fluid moves toward the area of the higher osmotic pressure in an attempt to dilute the osmotic concentration.

Blood pressure, or capillary hydrostatic pressure, is not constant; as discussed earlier, it varies according to the arterial pressure, the venous pressure, and the precapillary and postcapillary resistances. An elevated arterial or venous pressure increases capillary hydrostatic pressure, as does an increase in venous (postcapillary) resistance. An increase in arteriolar resistance, closure of precapillary sphincters, or a decrease in arterial or venous pressure reduces the hydrostatic pressure in the capillary. The average capillary hydrostatic pressure ($P_c$) is approximately 25 mm Hg at the arterial end of the capillary and 10 mm Hg at the venous end. These values are lower in the head, when it is in the upright position, and higher in the lower extremities. The mean value between the arterial and venous ends of the capillary is approximately 17 mm Hg, which has been described as the normal functional mean capillary pressure.[49]

Tissue pressure, or interstitial hydrostatic pressure ($P_i$), opposes capillary filtration, and the difference between the two ($P_c - P_i$) constitutes the driving force for filtration. Measurement of a true tissue pressure is difficult, but is thought to be approximately $-6$ mm Hg. If this value is correct, the hydrostatic driving force for filtration [17 − (−6) = 23] is greater than the capillary hydrostatic pressure, thus favoring filtration of fluid out of the vessel.

The major obstacle to fluid loss from the capillaries is the osmotic pressure of the plasma protein, also known as colloid osmotic pressure and oncotic pressure ($\pi_p$). The normal human plasma colloid osmotic pressure averages approximately 28 mm Hg. This pressure tends to draw fluid into the capillary.

Even though most protein particles are prevented from passing through the capillary membrane because of their size, a few do leak through the pores into the interstitial space. These protein molecules create an interstitial fluid colloid osmotic pressure ($\pi_i$) of approximately 5 mm Hg. This pressure plays a small role in driving fluid out of the vessel.

The Starling hypothesis describes the relationship between colloid osmotic pressure and hydrostatic pressure and the role of these forces in regulating fluid passage across the capillary membrane. This hypothesis can be expressed by the equation

$$\text{Fluid movement} = k[(P_c + \pi_i) - (P_i + \pi_p)]$$

where $k$ represents the filtration constant for the capillary membrane, which is dependent on the specific permeability of the capillary and the capillary surface area perfused. Filtration, or fluid movement out of the vessel, occurs when the algebraic sum in this equation is positive. Absorption, or movement of fluid into the vessel, occurs when the algebraic sum is negative.

If numerical values are put into the formula, it can be seen that there is nearly an equilibrium between movement of fluid into and out of the vessel:

$$\begin{aligned} \text{Fluid movement} &= k[(17+5) - (-7+28)] \\ &= k[(22) - (21)] \\ &= k \times 1 \end{aligned}$$

However, there is a slight excess of filtration, known as net filtration, which is balanced by fluid return to the circulation through the lymphatics. The normal rate of net filtration for the entire body is approximately 1.7 to 3.5 ml/min. This value also represents the rate of fluid flow into the lymphatics each minute.

**Edema.** Derived from the Greek word meaning tumor or swelling, the term *edema* describes a collection of interstitial fluid that distends the tissues. Edema develops when the filtration-absorption relationship is disturbed and the rate at which interstitial fluid forms is faster than the rate at which it can be removed by capillary reabsorption or lymph drainage. There are four causes of edema: (1) increased capillary hydrostatic pressure, (2) decreased capillary colloid osmotic pressure, (3) blockage of the lymphatic system, and (4) increased capillary permeability.

Any clinical condition that causes either venous obstruction or arteriolar dilation can increase capillary hydrostatic pressure. For example, cardiac failure commonly causes increased capillary hydrostatic pressure. Decreased capillary colloid osmotic pressure results from conditions that reduce the quantity of protein in the plasma. Such clinical conditions include severe burns, nephrosis, and insufficient dietary protein intake. The lymphatic system can be obstructed as a result of surgical procedures for removal of cancerous tissue. Conditions that allow protein to pass easily through the capillary membrane include burns and allergic reactions. In the lung, increased permeability may occur with adult respiratory distress syndrome.

## Capacitance Vessels

As a result of its anatomical structure, the venous network is a distensible system that, together with the right atrium, the pulmonary circulation, and the left atrium, contains 85 percent of the total blood volume. Known as the capacitance vessels, the veins serve as a reservoir of variable capacity. Their compliance is approximately 30 times greater than that of the arterial network. (See Systemic Influences on Cardiac Output.)

## Pulmonary Vessels

The function of the pulmonary vessels is to transport venous blood from the right ventricle to the alveolar capillaries, where oxygen is obtained and carbon dioxide released, and to return oxygenated blood to the left atrium. To accomplish this, 100 percent of the blood volume passes through the lungs: 98 percent via the pulmonary artery and 2 percent via the bronchial arteries. As noted earlier, the volume of blood ejected per stroke into the pulmonary circulation is virtually equal to the volume ejected per stroke into the systemic circulation. The capacity of the pulmonary vessels is only 10 percent of the capacity of the systemic circulation, however. Only because of their anatomical design (i.e., short, thin-walled, compliant vessels) are the pulmonary vessels able to accommodate the volume and provide for gas exchange in the short time available between cardiac cycles.

**Pressure, Resistance, and Flow.** The normal mean pulmonary artery pressure is approximately 15 mm Hg, and the normal mean pulmonary capillary pressure is approximately 10 mm Hg. The mean pulmonary venous and left atrial pressure is approximately 5 mm Hg. Consequently, the gradient between the pulmonary artery and the capillary pressures equals the gradient between the capillary and pulmonary venous pressures, and the arterial and venous segments contribute equally to pulmonary vascular resistance. This is very different from the contributions made by comparable segments to the systemic vascular resistance.

Although the mean pressures presented are accurate at the level of the heart, these pressures are not representative of all pressures in the lung of an upright individual. In this individual, the pressure in the apex may be as low as $-2$ or $-3$ mm Hg and as high as 24 or 25 mm Hg at the base. The exact value varies according to the distance that the portion of the lung in question is from the heart (Figure 1–24). These pressure variations are important because of their influence on blood flow throughout the lung.

According to the simplified version of Poiseuille's equation, $Q = \Delta P/R$, flow is a factor of the pressure gradient and resistance. In the lung, the resistance of the vessels is influenced by the balance between the capillary pressure, which tends to distend the vessel, and the alveolar pressure, which opposes capillary distention. In the apex of an upright lung, the capillary pressure may be less than the alveolar pressure, resulting in the collapse of the vessel and, consequently, no flow to that portion of the lung. Conversely, capillary pressure at the base of the upright lung greatly exceeds alveolar pressure, resulting in dilation and increased flow. For this reason, pulmonary edema is first detected in the bottom of the lung, where the hydrostatic pressures are greater. In the midportion of the lung, arterial pressure exceeds alveolar pressure, but alveolar pressure may be higher than venous pressure; therefore, the venous resistance is increased, but the vessel is not

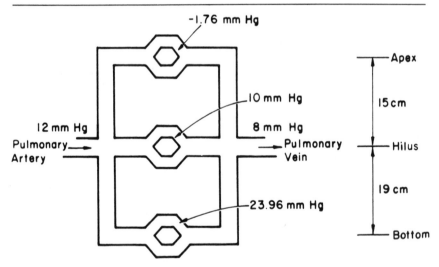

**Figure 1–24** Schematic diagram of the lung in the upright position. The capillary pressure at the heart level (hilus of the lung) is 10 mm Hg. This pressure becomes $-1.76$ mm Hg at the apex of the lung if it is 15 cm above the hilus and 23.96 mm Hg at the bottom of the lung if it is 19 cm below the hilus.

occluded and flow can occur. When the lung is in the supine position, the capillary pressures throughout the lung are similar, and the entire lung reacts much like the midportion of the upright lung.

Pulmonary vascular resistance is also influenced by the autonomic nervous system. Large and medium arterioles are innervated by both sympathetic and parasympathetic fibers. The vessels respond to α-stimulation by vasoconstricting, to β- and cholinergic-stimulation by vasodilating. Intrapulmonary veins and venules apparently are without autonomic innervation.

Another potent stimulus for increased pulmonary resistance is hypoxia. A local reduction in alveolar $Po_2$ produces vasoconstriction of the pulmonary vessels in that area. Systemic hypoxemia produces peripheral pulmonary vasodilation and a minor degree of generalized pulmonary vasoconstriction. This response by the pulmonary vessels to low alveolar oxygen pressure is a protective mechanism designed to shunt blood to the areas with greater oxygen concentration, thus maintaining adequate arterial and tissue oxygenation.

**Pulmonary Edema.** Under normal circumstances, the capillary hydrostatic pressure in the lung is 6 to 15 mm Hg, considerably lower than the colloid osmotic pressure of 28 mm Hg. Consequently, filtration does not usually occur in the alveolar-capillary bed, and the net inward-directed force promotes absorption of fluid. In addition, lympathic flow in the lungs is greater than that in other body parts. These two factors operate together to prevent fluid shifts into the alveoli. When the capillary hydrostatic pressure exceeds the colloid osmotic pressure or when filtration exceeds reabsorption and lymphatic drainage, however, pulmonary edema may result.

Pulmonary edema is a pathological state in which an abnormal amount of water is stored in the lungs. Not only do the tissues swell with fluid, creating interstitial edema, but also the fluid often replaces air, resulting in alveolar edema. The effects of pulmonary edema are

1. decreased lung compliance
2. increased airway resistance
3. increased work of breathing
4. abnormal perfusion, ventilation, and ventilation-perfusion balance
5. impaired gas exchange

Pulmonary edema may be classified as cardiogenic and noncardiogenic. Cardiogenic pulmonary edema results from increased pulmonary capillary hydrostatic pressure. Clinical conditions that precipitate increased capillary pressure include

• myocardial infarction
• arrhythmias

- cardiomyopathy
- hypertensive crisis
- volume overload secondary to blood transfusions or excessive infusion of intravenous fluids
- valvular lesions on the left side of the heart
- excessive exercise
- increased salt intake
- pregnancy
- anemia
- thyrotoxicosis

Noncardiogenic pulmonary edema results from increased permeability of the pulmonary capillary membrane (most commonly caused by acute respiratory distress syndrome) or from severe trauma to the central nervous system (neurogenic pulmonary edema). Acute respiratory distress syndrome may be secondary to shock, infections, trauma, liquid aspiration, drug ingestion, inhalation of toxins, hematologic disorders, and metabolic disorders. Neurogenic pulmonary edema may result from clinical conditions such as cerebral hemorrhage, stroke, tumors, and increased intracranial pressure.

## CARDIAC DYSFUNCTION

A number of clinical conditions produce the signs and symptoms of heart failure. It is important, however, to distinguish heart failure from either circulatory failure or myocardial failure. Heart failure is a clinical syndrome that is secondary to an alteration of the normal myocardial function; the heart loses its ability to pump blood adequately to meet the metabolic needs of the body. Heart failure occurs when the myocardium can no longer overcome a sustained hemodynamic overload, either a volume overload or a pressure overload. Lesions of the cardiac valves, systemic hypertension, pulmonary hypertension, and ischemic heart disease can cause such a hemodynamic overload.

The clinical picture of circulatory failure may resemble that of heart failure, even though cardiac function is normal or near normal. This form of failure may be known as high output failure. Conditions that lead to circulatory failure are renal disease, hepatic disease, anemia, and thyrotoxicosis.

Myocardial failure results from abnormalities in the contractile properties of the heart muscle. It is often difficult to determine the role of myocardial failure in the clinical syndrome of heart failure. It is apparent that primary myocardial failure (e.g., cardiomyopathy) often leads to heart failure and that primary cardiac defects (e.g., valvular lesions that result in heart failure) can and do cause some degree of myocardial failure.

## Compensatory Mechanisms for Heart Failure

The most common cause of cardiovascular dysfunction is prolonged hemodynamic overloading of the heart. Regardless of the cause, chronic hemodynamic overload activates a number of compensatory mechanisms. Some of these mechanisms are immediate responses to changes in volume or pressure load; others develop more slowly and progressively. They can be classified as cardiac compensatory mechanisms and extracardiac compensatory mechanisms.

The immediate cardiac compensatory mechanisms include the regulating mechanisms of preload, contractility, and heart rate, as discussed earlier. More long-term compensatory mechanisms within the heart are cardiac chamber dilation and hypertrophy of the cardiac cells. With chronic volume overload, the cardiac chambers stretch or dilate to accommodate the added volume. Because additional tension is required to maintain cardiac output under these circumstances, the cardiac cells increase in size (hypertrophy), resulting in an increased number of myofibrils and mitochondria; the cells do not increase in number, however.

Extracardiac compensatory mechanisms include those centered in the neural, adrenal, and renal systems. Stimulation of neural mechanisms increases sympathetic function and decreases parasympathetic function. As a result of sympathetic stimulation, the adrenal medulla secretes increased amounts of epinephrine and norepinephrine, thereby increasing the concentration of circulating catecholamines. Stimulation of the renal mechanisms results in retention of salt and water.

All these physiologic mechanisms are called into play in an attempt to maintain cardiac output and perfusion pressure in the presence of a dysfunctional cardiovascular system. Many of them place an added workload on the already failing heart, however. Without appropriate therapy, the heart eventually decompensates and cardiogenic shock and death may follow.

## Cardiovascular Decompensation

When preload is increased, whether because of decreased stroke volume or because of increased venous return, myocardial wall tension increases. This results in an increase in myocardial oxygen consumption. If the myocardial cells undergo hypertrophy in response to the increased wall tension, they require even more oxygen. Coronary circulation does not increase to match the increased myofibril and mitochondria formation, however. Consequently, oxygen supply does not equal oxygen demand, and cardiac performance further deteriorates.

Stimulation of carotid and aortic arch baroreceptors increases sympathetic stimulation to the myocardium and, thus, heart rate and contractility. Both of these alterations require increased oxygen. Over time, the coronary circulation cannot provide enough oxygen, the heart becomes ischemic, and failure ensues.

With sympathetic stimulation, peripheral arterioles constrict to maintain coronary and peripheral perfusion pressures. This vasoconstriction increases afterload, however. In turn, this increases the workload of the failing heart. Vasoconstriction also affects the circulating blood volume by reducing hydrostatic pressures and drawing interstitial fluids into the circulation. This increases preload, which again places additional work on the heart.

Reduced renal excretion of salt and water also affects circulating blood volume. Stimulation of the renin-angiotensin-aldosterone system not only leads to the reabsorption of sodium chloride and water, but also causes peripheral vasoconstriction, augmenting the sympathetic nervous system's vasoconstrictive effects. Hence, additional cardiac work is required to meet the demands of the increased preload and afterload.

Finally, when the heart fails, fluid backs up into the pulmonary system, increasing the capillary hydrostatic pressure in the pulmonary vasculature. When the forces promoting filtration exceed the forces promoting reabsorption, pulmonary edema occurs. Consequently, gas exchange is impaired and the oxygen content in the blood reduced. This further impairs the ability of the heart to extract the amount of oxygen that it needs to meet all its metabolic demands. Anaerobic metabolism thus leads to lactic acidosis, which further impairs the function of the myocardial cells.

Clearly, the system that begins as a positive feedback system for regulating and maintaining cardiac performance can become a negative feedback system that, without treatment, depletes the cardiac compensatory reserve. It is through appropriate hemodynamic monitoring and intervention that this downward decline in cardiac performance can be recognized and, it is hoped, halted.

---

NOTES

1. Thomas N. James et al., "Anatomy of the Heart," in *The Heart,* ed. J. Willis Hurst (New York: McGraw-Hill, 1982), 30.

2. Charles E. Rackley et al., "Tricuspid and Pulmonary Valve Disease," in *The Heart,* ed. J. Willis Hurst (New York: McGraw-Hill, 1982), 930.

3. Sandra L. Underhill, "Valvular Disorders," in *Cardiac Nursing,* ed. Sandra L. Underhill et al. (Philadelphia: J.B. Lippincott, 1982), 636.

4. James, "Anatomy of the Heart," 24–25.

5. Ibid., 25–26.

6. Ibid., 26.

7. Ibid., 32.

8. Ibid., 26.

9. Ibid., 27–28.

10. Robert F. Rushmer, *Structure and Function of the Cardiovascular System* (Philadelphia: W.B. Saunders, 1976), 135.

11. Ibid.

12. James, "Anatomy of the Heart," 34.

13. Ibid., 34–35.

14. Ibid., 35.

15. Ibid.

16. Ibid., 36.

17. Ibid., 47.

18. Ibid., 50–52.

19. Ibid., 52.

20. Carol Jean Halpenny, "Systemic and Pulmonary Circulations," in *Cardiac Nursing,* ed. Sandra L. Underhill et al. (Philadelphia: J.B. Lippincott, 1982), 47.

21. Ibid.

22. Ibid.

23. Arnold M. Katz, *Physiology of the Heart* (New York: Raven Press, 1977), 140.

24. Arthur C. Guyton, *Textbook of Medical Physiology* (Philadelphia: W.B. Saunders, 1981), 126.

25. Ibid.

26. Ibid., 126–127.

27. Ibid., 127.

28. Ibid., 153.

29. Ibid., 155.

30. Ibid.

31. Ibid.

32. Robert C. Schlant, Edmund H. Sonnenblick, and Richard Gorlin, "Normal Physiology of the Cardiovascular System," in *The Heart,* ed. J. Willis Hurst (New York: McGraw-Hill, 1982), 93.

33. James J. Smith and John P. Kampine, *Circulatory Physiology* (Baltimore: Williams & Wilkins, 1984), 100.

34. Ibid., 102.

35. Ibid.

36. Robert C. Little, *Physiology of the Heart and Circulation* (Chicago: Year Book Medical Publishers, 1985), 170.

37. J. Willis Hurst et al., "Atherosclerotic Coronary Heart Disease: Angina Pectoris, Myocardial Infarction, and Other Manifestations of Myocardial Ischemia," in *The Heart,* ed. J. Willis Hurst (New York: McGraw-Hill, 1982), 1118.

38. Guyton, *Textbook of Medical Physiology,* 170.

39. Ibid.

40. Ibid., 160.

41. John T. Shepherd and Paul M. Vanhoute, *The Human Cardiovascular System* (New York: Raven Press, 1979), 135.

42. Little, *Physiology of the Heart and Circulation,* 174.

43. Shepherd and Vanhoute, *Human Cardiovascular System,* 118.

44. Little, *Physiology of the Heart and Circulation,* 182.

45. Katz, *Physiology of the Heart,* 217.

46. Barry A. Shapiro, Ronald A. Harrison, and Carole A. Trout, *Clinical Application of Respiratory Care* (Chicago: Year Book Medical Publishers, 1975), 119.

47. Jacqueline F. Wade, *Respiratory Nursing Care* (St. Louis: C.V. Mosby, 1973), 52.

48. Smith and Kampine, *Circulatory Physiology,* 153.

49. Guyton, *Textbook of Medical Physiology,* 364.

# Chapter 2

# Monitoring Alterations in Cardiopulmonary Function

*Laura C. Young, R.N., M.S.N.*

Recognition of alterations in hemodynamics (the interrelationships of blood flow and the factors that influence it) and the proper interpretation of those alterations can determine the diagnosis, as well as the medical and nursing management of the patient. A full understanding of general hemodynamic principles, including those related to blood flow, the cardiac cycle, and oxygenation of the blood, is important to ensure an accurate interpretation of parameters.

## MEASUREMENT AND INTERPRETATION OF MONITORED PARAMETERS

### Relationship of Normal Waveform to Components of Cardiac Cycle

The relationship of the electrical activity to the mechanical activity of the heart is determined by factors such as cardiac innervation, autoregulation, electrolyte balance, anatomical structure, and pressure changes within the heart related to wall tension, vascular resistance, blood volume, and valve function. The waveforms of the various pressures measured in the assessment of hemodynamics can be correlated to the electrical activity of the heart, to cardiac valve closure, to contraction and relaxation of the cardiac chambers, and to the blood volume within the cardiac chambers (Figure 2–1).

*Correlation of Waveform Components*

Beginning with ventricular systole, which is initiated in the isometric contraction phase, the peak of the R wave on the electrocardiogram (ECG) and the closure of the atrioventricular valves coincide. This produces $S_1$, the first heart sound. The semilunar valves remain closed during this phase, and the ventricular pressures begin to rise above the atrial pressures. They continue to rise rapidly, until they

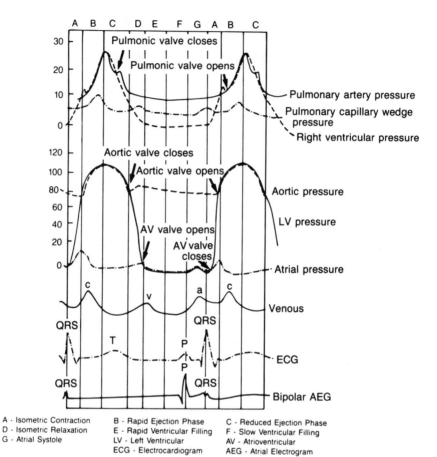

**Figure 2–1** Pressure waveforms correlated to electrical activity, valve state, contraction, and volume.

exceed aortic pressure (or afterload). Muscle fibers do not shorten and blood is not ejected early in systole, because all the valves are closed. Only when ventricular pressures exceed aortic and pulmonary pressures can ejection occur.

When the semilunar valves open and the external muscle fibers shorten, blood is ejected very rapidly from the ventricles at first (i.e., during the rapid ejection phase). The opening of the pulmonic valve during this phase produces the characteristic notch on the upstroke of the right ventricular pressure waveform, because the right ventricular pressure drops briefly as blood moves into the pulmonary artery. A rapid rise in aortic pressure and a sudden reduction in ventricular blood volume result. The c wave on the venous pressure tracing occurs during this phase as a result of the closure of the atrioventricular valves during ventricular contraction (see Figure 2–1). This phase corresponds to the ST segment of the ECG.

The second part of the ejection phase, called the reduced ejection phase, occurs as the expulsion of ventricular blood slows. Aortic pressure decreases, and the semilunar valves close. This phase correlates well with the T wave or ventricular repolarization on the ECG. It is also during this phase that the characteristic notch in the pulmonary artery pressure waveform appears on downstroke; this is directly related to closure of the pulmonic valve. Closure of the aortic valve at the end of this phase produces the incisura, which results from a transient backflow of blood as the ventricles begin to relax and aortic pressure drops slightly. The second heart sound, $S_2$, is produced by closure of the aortic valve. A residual volume of blood remains in the ventricles at the end of this phase.

The following phase, isometric relaxation, is characterized by several factors. The pressure returns to normal diastolic pressure. The ECG returns to baseline. The ventricle is relaxed, and all valves are closed. There is no change in ventricular blood volume during this phase, but the ventricular pressures fall rapidly below aortic and pulmonary artery pressures—they remain higher than atrial pressures, however. A corresponding delayed rise occurs in venous pressure from the previous closure of the atrioventricular valves and the backward bulge into the atrium that occurred in the isometric contraction phase. This produces the beginning of the v wave of the venous waveform.

When the ventricular pressure falls below the atrial pressure, the atrioventricular valves open, and a large volume of blood moves from the atria to the ventricles. During this rapid ventricular filling phase, the major portion of blood volume moves into the ventricle because of the pressure gradient.

Little change occurs during the slow ventricular filling phase, which follows. Very little additional blood volume moves during this time. The beginning of atrial depolarization, or the P wave, begins during this phase.

Atrial systole, the last phase of ventricular diastole, contributes 25 to 30 percent of ventricular volume. It begins with the peak of the P wave and continues until atrial pressure again drops as ventricular filling ends. The venous a wave appears during this phase of the cardiac cycle and is related to atrial contraction.

The bipolar atrial electrogram (AEG) provides additional information in relation to electrical activity (see Figure 2–1). The characteristic pattern for the atrial electrogram, used with cardiac surgery patients, corresponds to the usual ECG pattern throughout the cardiac cycle. It can distinguish atrial arrhythmias that are masked on ECG.

*Pressure Characteristics*

Three positive deflections occur in the atrial waveforms during each cardiac cycle. One is associated with atrial systole or contraction. The second is a result of closure of the atrioventricular valves. The third, larger positive deflection occurs when the ventricles are bulging and pressure in the ventricles is rising. The bulging of the atrioventricular valves back into the atria during this phase increases the pressure within the atria, thus producing the third positive deflection.

Ventricular pressures reach much higher peaks than atrial pressures. The ventricular waveform generated in each cardiac cycle differs from the atrial waveform in several ways. For example, it has only one positive deflection, and this deflection is significantly larger than either atrial deflection. The diastolic pressure of the ventricle is essentially equal to the diastolic pressure of the atrium.

Aortic pressure differs from both the ventricular and atrial pressures in its characteristics. The diastolic component of the aortic waveform is at a higher pressure than either the atrial or the ventricular diastolic pressure. The ventricular systolic pressure only slightly exceeds the aortic systolic pressure so that the two pressure waveforms nearly coincide. The aortic pressure waveform, however, has the characteristic incisura that appears when ventricular relaxation begins and the aortic valve closes.

The pulmonary artery pressure waveform is similar to the pressure waveform of the right ventricle. Both are low-pressure waveforms, but closure of the pulmonic valve produces a higher diastolic pressure in the pulmonary artery than in the right ventricle. Diastolic pressure in the right ventricle continues to drop after closure of the valve.

The pulmonary capillary wedge pressure is a measurement obtained by means of a balloon-tipped catheter placed in the pulmonary artery. Because there is normally no obstruction between the left atrium and the pulmonary artery, the arterial pressure measurement is equal to the left atrial pressure. During diastole, when the mitral valve is open, the pulmonary artery pressure should also equal left ventricular end-diastolic pressure.

## Direct Hemodynamic Parameters

Catheters of various sizes and complexity are used to measure the parameters of cardiopulmonary function. Each parameter has its normal limits (Table 2–1) and may be altered by various means. Knowledge of the relationship of these parameters to the total clinical picture is essential for accurate diagnosis and intervention.

### Central Venous Pressure

In the past, central venous pressure (CVP) was used as an indication of left ventricular function. The right and left sides of the heart function somewhat independently, however, and CVP is a measure of right atrial pressure. Moreover, right atrial pressure reflects primarily right ventricular end-diastolic pressure. If

**Table 2–1** Normal Range for Cardiopulmonary Pressures

| Pressure | Acronym | Normal Range |
|---|---|---|
| Central venous pressure | CVP | 4–15 cm $H_2O$, 3–11 mm Hg |
| Right atrial pressure | RAP | 2–6 mm Hg |
| Right ventricular systolic pressure | RVS | 20–30 mm Hg |
| Right ventricular diastolic pressure | RVD | 0–5 mm Hg |
| Pulmonary artery systolic pressure | PAS | 20–30 mm Hg |
| Pulmonary artery diastolic pressure | PAD | 10–20 mm Hg |
| Pulmonary artery mean pressure | PAM | 10–15 mm Hg |
| Pulmonary capillary wedge pressure | PCWP | 4–12 mm Hg |
| Left atrial pressure | LAP | 4–12 mm Hg |
| Left ventricular systolic pressure | LVS | 100–140 mm Hg |
| Left ventricular diastolic pressure | LVD (LVEDP) | 5–12 mm Hg |
| Aortic systolic pressure | AoS | 100–140 mm Hg |
| Aortic diastolic pressure | AoD | 60–80 mm Hg |
| Aortic mean pressure | AoM (MAP) | 70–90 mm Hg |

right and left ventricular end-diastolic pressures were similar, and if changes in these pressures occurred simultaneously, CVP would reflect left ventricular function. Unfortunately, this is not the case. Selective depression of either ventricle, which frequently occurs with ischemic heart disease or pulmonary disease, has a totally different effect on each side. Thus, while CVP is valuable in monitoring blood volume and venous return, it has little value in monitoring cardiovascular status.

Central venous pressure may be estimated or measured directly. If there is no obstruction between the right atrium and the neck veins, CVP can be estimated noninvasively through observation of the neck veins. In estimating CVP, these steps must be followed:

1. Identify the approximate location of the right atrium (phlebostatic level) on the chest. Mark this location for future comparative measurements.
2. Raise the patient's head to a semi-Fowler's position. Note whether the measurement is taken with the patient's bed at an angle of 30°, 45°, etc. for comparison. If necessary for patient comfort, the head may be elevated to an angle of 90°.
3. Examine the neck veins for distention of the jugular veins. Watch carefully when the patient breathes deeply for a drop in venous distention. Raising or lowering the head of the bed somewhat may decrease or increase distention, respectively. All measurements taken for comparison must be at the same level.
4. Identify the top level of distention. Identify the middle of the right atrium.

5. Measure the vertical distance between these two points with a ruler graduated in centimeters. This is the estimated CVP.

In some patients, it is difficult or impossible to estimate CVP by this method. Problems that may lead to an inaccurate CVP estimate are

- marked distention of the veins as a result of local venous distention or very high venous pressures
- inability to locate veins
- inability to elevate head
- no noticeable distention

Occasionally, an inexperienced examiner may confuse arterial pulsations with venous pulsations.

Central venous pressure is directly measured through percutaneous placement of a CVP catheter in the superior vena cava. Once the line has been placed and secured, pressure can be measured continuously through the use of a pressure transducer or manual use of a manometer. Accuracy in measurement and consistency in comparison are important. Identification of the phlebostatic level at which all measurements are taken and assurance that the patient's head is at the same level for each measurement are essential for accurate results. Ventilator distortion of pressures related to changes in intrathoracic pressures may cause inaccuracies in patients who require assisted ventilation.

Examination of the venous waveform reveals three deflections (see Figure 2–1). Each wave deflection can be correlated to activity in the cardiac cycle. Atrial contraction during diastole increases the atrial pressure, resulting in the venous a wave. The x descent occurs as the atrial pressure drops. When the atrioventricular valves close, the c wave appears. The v wave for the venous pulse occurs just before the atrioventricular valves open, and is followed by sudden reduction in pressure (y descent) when the valves open and blood passively rushes into the ventricles.[1]

In the interpretation of CVP measurements, several principles must be remembered. Measurements obtained manually with a manometer are usually given in centimeters of water. They should not be compared to measurements obtained from a transducer, which are usually given in millimeters of mercury, unless the pressures are converted to the same scale. Mercury is 13.6 times as heavy as water; therefore, 1 mm Hg converts to 13.6 mm or 1.36 cm $H_2O$. To convert centimeters of water to millimeters of mercury, it is necessary to divide the number of centimeters of water by 1.36.

Although the normal range of CVP values is 4 to 15 cm $H_2O$, emphasis should be placed on the patient's individual normal value. Trends are more significant than are single values. Most important, a normal CVP does not necessarily indicate normal circulatory function or the absence of disease.

Correct placement of the central venous catheter is obviously important and can be confirmed only through roentgenogram.[2] The catheter may be malpositioned at insertion, or it may migrate with patient movement. Complications associated with malposition include cardiac perforation and damage to the pulmonary artery, as well as inaccurate readings. The fluid level may fluctuate in incorrectly placed catheters, also producing inaccurate readings. In light of the potential inaccuracies and the normal readings frequently noted in the presence of significantly abnormal cardiovascular function, CVP should not be relied on as the only parameter to determine hemodynamic status.

Several physiologic abnormalities may cause an elevation in CVP. Increased preload related to fluid overload, fluid retention, valvular insufficiency, and left-to-right shunting in the heart may cause an elevated CVP. Chronic renal or cardiac failure that produces fluid retention and excessive intravenous intake of fluids may increase preload, elevating CVP. A ventricular septal defect may cause the left-to-right cardiac shunt associated with the elevated CVP from increased preload. Constrictive pericarditis, right ventricular infarction, and myocarditis adversely affect contractility and increase CVP.

An increase in afterload of the right ventricle or a reduction in right ventricular contractility may also increase CVP. A variety of disease states may cause these physiologic abnormalities. Chronic obstructive pulmonary disease, pulmonic stenosis, or pulmonary embolus, for instance, increase the right ventricular afterload. Pulmonary hypertension may also increase this afterload, but it is often related to other disorders.

Inadequate venous return may be related to several abnormalities and results in a reduced CVP. Hypovolemia from blood loss or water excretion in exercise reduces venous return. Excessive vasodilation or venodilation reduces the circulating blood volume and CVP.

### Arterial Pressure

Fluctuating between the lower diastolic and higher systolic pressures, arterial pressure is at its highest point in the aorta. As blood traverses the circulatory system, the pressure drops. The drop in pressure is related to the resistance to flow in the system. Through hydraulic filtering, the circulatory system is able to maintain a somewhat constant pressure throughout the cardiac cycle and a steady rather than intermittent flow to the capillaries.

Blood moves from the aorta, where it meets resistance, back to the right atrium, where it meets no resistance. Variations in resistance in the circulatory system produce variations in mean arterial pressure and variations in the contour of the waveform (Figure 2–2). These waveforms correlate to the aortic valve opening in slightly different ways.

The aortic pressure pulse wave is very similar to the carotid pressure pulse wave. It characteristically rises rapidly during systole, then more slowly until it reaches its peak. As the pressure falls, the wave is interrupted by the incisura, which occurs after closure of the aortic valve; the backflow of blood into the aortic root that follows this valve's closure increases the pressure slightly, creating the incisura in the pressure curve. Pressure then drops quickly and slows the peripheral runoff.

The more distant the artery from the heart, the more significant the change in the waveform. Characteristic changes include

- a delay in the rise in pressure in relation to the aortic valve opening
- a steeper upstroke of the curve

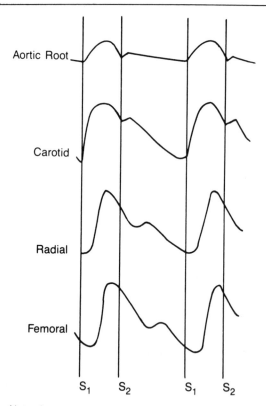

Note: S₁ - Aortic Valve opens. S₂ - Aortic Valve Closes.

**Figure 2–2** Arterial waveform variations. $S_1$, aortic valve opens; $S_2$, aortic valve closes.

- a narrower and more peaked curve
- replacement of the incisura with a dicrotic notch that appears lower on the curve[3]

Several other changes may occur in the waveform at the peripheral arteries. As the blood travels from one area to another, the waveform may taper as the wave is amplified; as the blood encounters resistance in the peripheral arterioles, however, damping of the waveform also occurs. The pulse pressure in the capillaries is nearly zero under normal conditions.

The mean arterial pressure (*MAP*) is determined by the following equation:

$$MAP = DP + 1/3 \, (SP - DP)$$

where *DP* is diastolic pressure and *SP* is systolic pressure. The mean arterial pressure is determined by both blood volume and the peripheral vascular resistance; like resistance, pressure varies from vessel to vessel. Pressure in the aorta is highest; it becomes progressively lower as blood passes from the aorta to arteries to arterioles and capillaries. When blood returns to the right atrium, it meets no resistance, and the right atrial pressure approaches zero (normal, 2 to 6 mm Hg).

Arterial pressure may be measured in several ways. For example, it may be measured with a sphygmomanometer, or it may be measured directly with an arterial line and transducer. As with the CVP catheter, correct placement of the lines is important for accuracy. Patient movement, arterial catheter obstruction, or even placement of the catheter against the vessel wall can affect the pressure reading obtained when arterial lines are used, making the result inaccurate. Patient movement can affect the reading of manual sphygmomanometers as well. Because the use of a cuff that is too large or too small may affect pressure readings, the use of cuffs that are especially designed for children or obese patients, as indicated, improves accuracy significantly. As with any equipment, calibration and appropriate zero balance are important.

The causes for variations in arterial blood pressure are numerous. They range from pathological conditions of various body organs to stress or anxiety (the psychophysiologic stress response). For example, pulse pressure increases with an increase in stroke volume. Whenever stroke volume increases, the greater volume of blood ejected with each contraction must be spread throughout the arterial system. The pressure rises in systole, which results in a larger fall of the diastolic pressure. Hypervolemia, some bradycardias, and aortic regurgitation increase the stroke volume and pulse pressure.

Some drugs (e.g., isoproterenol, dopamine, and dobutamine) increase pulse pressure by increasing the ventricular ejection velocity. When blood is forced from the ventricle at such a rapid rate, there is no time for peripheral runoff to keep the arterial pressure down. The aortic pressure rises rapidly, with an associated elevation in pulse pressure.

Decreased arterial compliance occurs in patients with hypertension. This increases pulse pressure because the arterioles can accommodate less blood. Vessels that have become rigid with arteriosclerosis lose their elasticity and their compliance, also leading to a rise in pulse pressure.

Peripheral vascular resistance also plays a role in the elevation of pulse pressure. When the peripheral vascular resistance is reduced, blood flows rapidly from the arterioles to the veins. This increases venous return to the heart, filling pressures, and stroke volume. The subsequent reduction in afterload also reduces cardiac work. Several conditions decrease peripheral vascular resistance—hyperthyroidism, fever, anemia, and exercise.

A reduction in stroke volume decreases the rise in pressure during systole and, therefore, the pulse pressure. Shock and heart failure reduce stroke volume. Because an increase in afterload also reduces the volume of each ejection, conditions that increase peripheral vascular resistance and, thus, afterload (e.g., shock, metabolic acidosis, severe cold, or an increased level of norepinephrine) reduce pulse pressure.

Prolongation of ejection time is another mechanism that reduces pulse pressure. Aortic stenosis prolongs ejection time, for example, allowing time for peripheral runoff during systole.

Pressures within specific vessels are frequently related to vessel abnormalities. Coarctation of the aorta may produce elevated pressures in the arteries of the upper extremities and head, while pressures below the coarctation remain normal or low. Similarly, pressures behind stenoses are elevated, while those beyond the point of stenosis are low or normal. Stenosis of the renal artery may result in a systemic hypertension, because the low pressure within the kidney may initiate the compensatory response of the renin-angiotensin system to elevate a pressure that, in reality, does not need to be increased.

*Intracardiac Pressure*

Each chamber of the heart has a different pressure (see Table 2–1), and the waveform of each chamber differs from that of the others. As with all cardiac pressures, pressure in one chamber must rise above the pressure in the next chamber to allow opening of valves and movement of blood from an area of greater pressure to an area of lesser pressure. The right atrial pressure waveform is very similar to the CVP waveform. It has three positive deflections that may be identical to the CVP deflections. The correlation of the right atrial pressure waveform to those of the ECG, atrial electrogram, and valve function may be seen in Figure 2–1. The a wave corresponds to the PR segment of the ECG. The RST junction on the ECG corresponds to the c wave, and the v wave corresponds to the T-P timing on the ECG. The right atrial pressure may be altered by various disease states.

The right ventricular pressure waveform occurs in two phases. The first phase, the isometric contraction, occurs after the tricuspid valve closes and before the pulmonic valve opens. In this phase, pressure rises as the right ventricle contracts in a closed chamber filled with a volume of blood. When the pressure exceeds the pulmonary artery pressure, the pulmonic valve opens, and the right ventricular pressure drops as the right ventricle empties. This phase is called the ejection phase. When the ventricle empties and the pulmonic valve closes, the pressure that occurs with backward flow against the closed pulmonic valve causes a dicrotic notch on the pulmonary arterial waveform (see Figure 2–1). The ejection phase of the right ventricle generally corresponds to the QT interval on the ECG.

During relaxation of the ventricle, diastole, the ventricle fills with blood from the right atrium, with a corresponding increase in pressure. End-diastolic pressure is measured just before systole occurs, corresponding to the QT interval on the ECG.

Abnormalities in the filling of the right ventricle or ejection from the right ventricle can result in abnormal measurements of right ventricular pressure. During pulmonary artery pressure monitoring, it is important to observe the waveform, because the pulmonary artery catheter may move backward into the right ventricle, thus changing the waveform.

The left atrial pressure waveform corresponds to the left ventricular end-diastolic pressure, pulmonary artery end-diastolic pressure, and pulmonary capillary wedge pressure. At specific points in the cardiac cycle, when the mitral valve is open, there is normally no barrier between the pulmonary artery and the left ventricle. The pressures equilibrate throughout the system (Figure 2–3). The left ventricle fills with blood from the left atrium so that the left chambers are briefly one chamber. Because there are no valves between the pulmonary artery and the

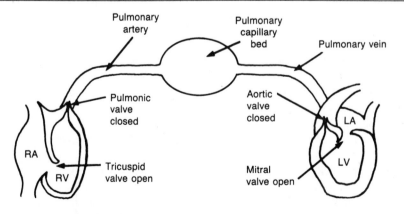

**Figure 2–3** Equalization of pulmonary artery and left heart pressures. *RA,* right atrium; *RV,* right ventricle; *LA,* left atrium; *LV,* left ventricle.

left atrium, the area from the closed pulmonic to the closed aortic valve temporarily becomes a closed system. If the patient has either pulmonary disease or mitral valve disease, however, this does not occur; such disease creates barriers to blood flow and equilibration of pressures.

Intracardiac pressures may be measured directly or indirectly. A flow-directed balloon-tipped catheter may be used in the direct measurement of right pressures and indirect measurement of left pressures. Such a catheter is placed by a physician, and correct placement is essential. Proper positioning is confirmed by waveform patterns and/or roentgenogram. These catheters are useful to the critical care nurse in obtaining data related to intracardiac parameters.

Partial occlusion of the catheter or placement against the vessel wall can dampen the waveform and produce inaccurate results. Patient position, previously believed to be extremely important in the measurement of intracardiac pressures, has been shown to be less important. Placement of the transducer at heart level, however, is essential to accuracy. Patient movement and deep ventilation may also influence readings. Positive pressure ventilation can affect venous return, therefore influencing intracardiac pressures. For these reasons, care must be taken to ensure proper catheter placement and transducer position. Patient movement during pressure measurement should be minimized and ventilation controlled as much as possible. Removal of the patient from mechanical ventilation is helpful in obtaining accurate readings, but this is not always feasible.

Right atrial pressure corresponds to CVP. Those conditions that elevate CVP (e.g., right ventricular failure, pulmonary hypertension, fluid overload, chronic obstructive pulmonary disease, and pulmonic stenosis) also elevate right atrial pressure. Inadequate venous return reduces both right atrial pressure and CVP. The hypovolemia or excessive vasodilation that causes a low venous return results not only in a low CVP, but also in a low right atrial pressure. (For a discussion of measurement, see Central Venous Pressure.)

Right ventricular pressure is elevated when there is an increased afterload. Pulmonic stenosis and pulmonary hypertension increase afterload and, thus, right ventricular pressure. A ventricular septal defect with shunting of blood from left to right in the heart or fluid overload increases the right ventricular preload and pressure. Such conditions as right ventricular infarct, constrictive pericarditis, and myocarditis of the right ventricle reduce contractility and increase right ventricular pressure.

Low right ventricular pressures are normal, but an abnormally low right ventricular pressure may occur when right ventricular preload is reduced. In hypovolemic states that reduce venous return significantly, right ventricular pressures are abnormally low.

Left atrial pressure can be measured at the patient's bedside, although there is some danger of systemic embolization from air or clots. Left atrial pressure reflects the left ventricular end-diastolic pressure in the absence of mitral valve disease. It also correlates well with the pulmonary capillary wedge pressure within a range of 5 to 25 mm Hg. Above 25 mm Hg, the left atrial pressure tends to be higher than the pulmonary capillary wedge pressure.[4]

Left atrial pressure increases when the left ventricular preload is elevated, the left ventricular afterload is elevated, or left ventricular contractility is reduced. Insufficiency of the mitral valve may also increase left atrial pressure, because it may allow regurgitation from the left ventricle. Aortic insufficiency indirectly affects left atrial pressure as well. Reduced contractility of the left ventricle from infarction, cardiomyopathy, or left ventricular failure also increases left atrial pressure. Finally, increased afterload related to increased peripheral vascular resistance, aortic stenosis, or abnormalities (e.g., coarctation of the aorta) increase left atrial pressure.

A low left atrial pressure is generally related to reduced circulating volume. This may result from excessive vasodilation or from hypovolemia. The vasodilation may be physiologic or drug-induced.

Left ventricular end-diastolic pressure cannot be measured directly at the patient's bedside because of the danger of dysrhythmias and embolization. Elevation of left ventricular end-diastolic pressure is often associated with an elevated preload related to such conditions as aortic insufficiency or volume overload. Increased afterload as a result of increased peripheral vascular resistance, coarctation of the aorta, or aortic stenosis also increases left ventricular end-diastolic pressure. Most significant, however, are increases in left ventricular end-diastolic pressure related to conditions that decrease left ventricular compliance, such as left ventricular failure, myocardial infarction, and cardiomyopathies.

Like a low left atrial pressure, a low left ventricular end-diastolic pressure is associated with low preload or low afterload. These may be associated with low volume states (low preload) and reduced venous return, or with excessive vasodilation (low afterload).

*Pulmonary Artery Pressures*

Waveforms of pulmonary artery pressure can be divided into systolic and diastolic portions. A steep rise with ejection of blood from the right ventricle is the systolic portion. A slower decrease in pressure follows until the closure of the pulmonic valve produces the dicrotic notch on the waveform. Diastole begins at this point, and the measurement of pulmonary artery end-diastolic pressure is obtained at the end of the diastolic phase.

Pulmonary artery end-diastolic pressure correlates to pulmonary artery wedge pressure in the absence of pulmonary disease. Variations in pulmonary artery end-diastolic pressure can occur with changes in intrathoracic pressure during respiration, especially in patients who use a ventilator. The patient must breathe quietly if measurement of these pressures is to be accurate. If the patient is unable to control his or her breathing pattern, the pressure should be measured at end-expiration to ensure results that are as accurate as possible. Excessive catheter movement can alter readings, resulting in inaccurate measurement of the pressure. In addition, the presence of pulmonary disease or tachycardias greater than 125 beats/min must be considered in the measurement of pulmonary artery pressure as reflective of left ventricular end-diastolic pressure.[5]

Left atrial pressure (or left atrial filling pressure) and pulmonary capillary wedge pressure waveforms are similar in appearance to the right atrial waveform with a, c, and v waves. The a wave of the left atrial pressure follows the P wave on the ECG because of the slight delay in transmitting the pressure at the catheter tip to the transducer. When the mitral valve closes at the beginning of ventricular contraction, the c wave appears on the left atrial pressure tracing. As the ventricle contracts in late systole, bulging of the atrioventricular valve into the atrium produces the v wave. The c wave is usually not identified on the pulmonary capillary wedge tracing. The v wave correlates to the T wave or just after the T on the ECG. If the mitral valve is insufficient, the v wave is very high on the tracing.

Normally, there is a drop in pressure as the pulmonary artery catheter balloon is inflated to obtain the pulmonary capillary wedge pressure, as well as a rise in pressure as the balloon is deflated. If these changes are not noted, there may be a problem with the catheter that requires correction.

Several factors that must be considered in measurement of pulmonary artery, left atrial, and left ventricular pressures relate to the catheter itself. Damping of the waveform occurs if the tip is occluded or, occasionally, if the tip has been placed against the wall of the vessel. Air bubbles in the tubing or the catheter can also cause damping. Improper leveling of the transducer can contribute to inaccurate readings. Loose connections, catheter fling from turbulent blood flow, and migration of the catheter tip are other causes of inaccurate readings.

Although there has been a great deal of controversy surrounding the issue of the proper patient position for accurate measurement of pulmonary artery pressures, more recent studies support the belief that it is unnecessary to reposition patients for pulmonary artery pressure measurements.[6] It is important that transducer placement be appropriately aligned with the phlebostatic level, however. Failure to zero-balance, calibrate or place the transducer appropriately can also result in inaccuracies in pressure measurement.

Pulmonary artery end-diastolic pressure and pulmonary capillary wedge pressure correlate very well with left ventricular end-diastolic pressure. Reasons for elevations or reductions in these pressures are the same as those for left atrial pressure and left ventricular end-diastolic pressure. There are a few exceptions to direct correlation between pulmonary capillary wedge pressure, left atrial pressure, and left ventricular end-diastolic pressure.

There can be no obstruction between the pulmonary artery and the left ventricle if direct correlation among the pressures is to be assumed, as is the case when the pulmonary capillary wedge pressure is the only parameter monitored. Obstructions such as stenosis of the mitral valve, obstructive processes of the pulmonary venous system, or left atrial myxomas make correlations inaccurate. In the presence of these conditions or with high intra-alveolar pressure from positive pressure ventilation, the pulmonary capillary wedge pressure is higher than is the left ventricular end-diastolic pressure. When the compliance or contractility of the left ventricle is decreased (e.g., by tamponade, acute infarction, or left ventricular failure), the pulmonary capillary wedge pressure should be lower than is the actual left ventricular end-diastolic pressure. A high left ventricular end-diastolic pressure (greater than 25 mm Hg) is also not accurately reflected in the pulmonary capillary wedge pressure, which would be less.

Elevated pulmonary artery pressures may reflect increased pulmonary blood volume or increased pulmonary vascular resistance. Pulmonary embolism, pulmonary hypertension, or vasoconstriction of pulmonary vessels related to hypoxia or hypercapnia may increase pulmonary artery pressure. Low pulmonary artery pressures are, as indicated, related to hypovolemia (actual or relative).

*Cardiac Output*

Yet another parameter to be used in evaluating cardiopulmonary status is cardiac output. Because of the direct relationship between cardiac output and left ventricular performance, measurement of the cardiac output has proved quite valuable in the assessment of the response to intervention.

Defined as the amount of blood ejected by the heart within a specified time period (usually each minute), cardiac output can be measured in several ways. One method of determining cardiac output is the dye indicator dilution method. This method is rarely used at the patient's bedside, but it is commonly used in cardiac catheterization laboratories. It involves a dye or other easily detectable, water-soluble, nontoxic substance that will not be metabolized during the period in which the sample is to be taken. A dye frequently used for this procedure is indocyanine, also called cardiogreen. The concentration of this dye in the blood can be measured with a densitometer, an apparatus that determines the dye concentration spectrophotometrically over a time period.

A predetermined amount of the dye indicator is injected intravenously while arterial blood is withdrawn steadily through the densitometer. The densitometer records graphically the curve of dye concentration (Figure 2–4), and the cardiac output is then determined by a formula called the Stewart-Hamilton equation:

$$CO = \frac{I \times 60}{Cm \times t} \times \frac{1}{K}$$

where

$$CO = \text{cardiac output (liters/min)}$$
$$I = \text{dye injected (mg)}$$
$$60 = \text{seconds per minute}$$
$$Cm = \text{mean indicator concentration (mg/liter)}$$
$$t = \text{mean in seconds of total curve duration}$$
$$K = \text{calibration factor (mm deflection produced by known concentration of dye)}$$

The first denominator for the equation is the measurement of the area under the curve from the appearance of the dye until its disappearance. Unfortunately, the recirculation disrupts the curve on the down slope and may alter the accuracy of the calculation. Replotting the curve semilogarithmically improves accuracy, and the area under the curve can be measured by planimetry. The measurement can then be multiplied by the calibration factor to relate the curve height to dye concentration more accurately. The simplest way to determine the area under the curve is to use a computer.

This particular method is complicated by the need for connecting equipment: a pump for withdrawing arterial blood from a peripheral artery, a densitometer for recording the dye concentration, and a recorder to plot the curve. The use of a

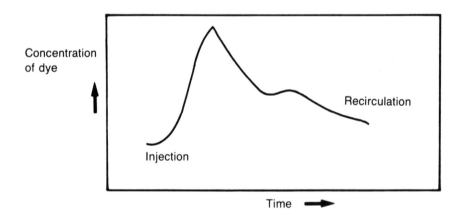

**Figure 2–4** Curve of dye concentration in dye indicator dilution method for determining cardiac output.

computer to determine the area under the curve adds another piece of equipment. Although the dye indicator dilution method has only a $\pm$ 5 percent error, readings are more accurate for measuring high cardiac outputs than for measuring low cardiac outputs.[7]

The thermodilution method for measuring cardiac output is most commonly used at the patient's bedside. In this technique, a solution with a known temperature is injected into the bloodstream, and the change in temperature is measured at a downstream site. The formula used to determine cardiac output is based on the premise that the heat gained by the fluid injected when it mixes with blood is equal to the heat lost by the blood. This technique gained popularity in the early 1970s because of its strong theoretical base and its strong correlation with dye-determined and heat-determined measurements.[8]

The Stewart-Hamilton equation must be modified to adjust for the specific gravity and the specific heat of both the blood and injectate, because the temperature change is affected by these variables. Because the temperature may increase as the injectate traverses the catheter, a correction factor must also be added. Thus, the formula used with the thermodilution method is

$$CO = \frac{V(T_B - T_I)}{A} \times \frac{(S_I)(C_I)}{(S_B)(C_B)} \times \frac{(60)(C)(K)}{1}$$

where

$$
\begin{aligned}
CO &= \text{cardiac output} \\
V &= \text{volume injected} \\
A &= \text{area under thermodilution curve} \\
T_B, T_I &= \text{temperature of blood and injectate} \\
S_B, S_I &= \text{specific gravity of blood and injectate} \\
C_B, C_I &= \text{specific heat of blood and injectate} \\
60 &= \text{seconds per minute} \\
C &= \text{correction factor} \\
K &= \text{calibration constant}
\end{aligned}
$$

Cardiac output can be determined by the thermodilution method with relative ease, repetitively and rapidly. Although there is some indication that measurements are more accurate when iced solutions are used, either iced or room temperature solutions are acceptable. A measured amount of cold fluid is injected into the right atrium through a right atrial line or the proximal lumen of a flow-directed, balloon-tipped catheter. Either the thermistor on the catheter tip or a separate thermistor catheter located in the pulmonary artery is used to detect the temperature change.

The use of a computer to perform the cardiac output calculation makes this method rather simple to employ. The volume of the injectate, the temperature of the blood and injectate, and the calibration factor are generally known or can be measured by the computer. All other parts of the equation are programmed into the computer or are calculated during injection. A thermodilution curve is recorded; this curve is similar to the dye dilution curve, except for the recirculation distortion.

The radioisotope and pulse contour methods of determining cardiac output are seldom used in the clinical setting. The radioisotope method, in which radioactive tracers are used, is more commonly used in conjunction with measurement of segmental wall motion. The pulse contour method, based on a formula that includes arterial pulse contour, relies on prior determination of the cardiac output by the Fick method:

$$CO = SV \times HR$$
$$SV = K \times (M - D)$$

where

$$
\begin{aligned}
CO &= \text{cardiac output} \\
SV &= \text{stroke volume} \\
HR &= \text{heart rate} \\
K &= \text{constant of pulse contour formula} \\
&\quad \text{obtained from initial determination of} \\
&\quad \text{cardiac output} \\
M &= \text{mean arterial pressure} \\
D &= \text{diastolic pressure}
\end{aligned}
$$

While the pulse contour method has some usefulness in monitoring stroke volume, it is not commonly used.

Cardiac output measurement, accomplished by any of the methods described, is quite accurate. There are several possible sources of error, however, and they must be considered before interventions are based on the measurement. With the dye indicator dilution method, errors may occur because of a prolonged injection time or a blood withdrawal rate that is not uniform. Dye that is old or does not mix well with the blood prior to the sample withdrawal alters results. (Because dye becomes unstable when exposed to light or over time, it should be freshly mixed each day.) Inaccurate measurement of the dye can produce errors in calculation, as can incomplete introduction of the dye into the circulation. An improperly calibrated instrument is another source of error. Furthermore, intracardiac shunts may distort the curve of the dye concentration, and the cardiac output measurement can be considered highly accurate under these circumstances.

The thermodilution method of cardiac output measurement has several advantages over the dye indicator dilution method. Because the indicator in the thermodilution method is the temperature of the injectate, not the concentration, there is no significant recirculation of the indicator. Therefore, serial cardiac output determinations may be performed as rapidly as every 45 to 60 seconds. The thermodilution method does not require withdrawal of blood, which eliminates the potential error associated with this procedure. Finally, the thermal curve calibration is quite easily performed.

Errors related to the thermodilution method are associated primarily with the improper location or position of the thermistor head or with improper injection technique. A thermistor that is too far advanced into a branch of the pulmonary artery or is against the vessel wall provides inaccurate cardiac output measurements. Volumes in the syringes of serial injections must be the same, and injections must be smooth and rapid; otherwise, errors occur. Some computers may even require automatic injection to ensure accuracy.

Another source of error is an undetected change in the injectate temperature, which may occur when the injectate has not cooled properly or when the syringe has been handled excessively. Delays in injection of the cooled solution through the catheter may also alter the calculation. Intracardiac shunts and severe disease of the pulmonic or tricuspid valves may distort the cardiac output measurement significantly.

Changes in cardiac output may be reflected in the serial cardiac output measurements. A change in the position of the patient or movement by the patient may alter the cardiac output by increasing venous return. Similarly, a change in the patient's temperature, heart rate, rhythm, or hemodynamic status may alter the cardiac output. Thus, serial measurements of cardiac output indicate any reduction in cardiac output and the degree of the heart's success in compensation. Both pieces of information are helpful in the diagnosis and selection of appropriate interventions.

Normal cardiac output measurements vary greatly from individual to individual because of wide variations in body size. While a cardiac output of 4.5 liters/min may be adequate for a small individual, a much larger cardiac output may be required to provide adequate tissue oxygenation in a 300-pound individual. A cardiac index, which is based on body surface area, is a more specific measurement. Cardiac index, or cardiac output per square meter of body surface area, has a normal range of 2.5 to 4 liters/min/m$^2$. The DuBois body surface chart may be used to determine the body surface area.[9]

### Hemoglobin Oxygen Saturation

Measurement of hemoglobin oxygen saturation may offer clues to the proper diagnosis and treatment of cardiopulmonary disease. The saturation of the hemoglobin with oxygen is expressed as the percentage of oxygen ($O_2$) that the hemoglobin carries in relation to the amount that it is potentially able to carry. The normal oxygen saturation varies according to the vessel from which the blood is taken. The saturation of blood drawn from tissue capillaries is low, because the oxygen has been extracted for use by the tissues. Arterial saturation, however, is expected to be high (i.e., 95 to 100 percent).

The relationship of oxygen saturation to the partial pressure of oxygen ($Po_2$) is characterized by the oxyhemoglobin dissociation curve (see Figure 1–22). As the $Po_2$ increases, the saturation increases, but it reaches a plateau at approximately 100 mm Hg. At this point, hemoglobin is 100 percent saturated. Increasing the $Po_2$ above 100 mm Hg does not improve saturation, as the hemoglobin is already carrying as much oxygen as possible. Even when the $Po_2$ is much lower, the saturation remains quite high. There is an 89 percent saturation, for instance, at a $Po_2$ of 60 mm Hg.

As blood traverses the tissue capillaries, oxygen is extracted from hemoglobin at a high rate, as shown by a steep decline on the oxyhemoglobin dissociation curve, without a significant decline in the $Po_2$. The amount of oxygen removed and the rate at which it is removed largely depend on the requirement of the tissue for oxygen. Certain tissues, such as the heart muscle, normally require more oxygen. The normal saturation of mixed venous blood returning to the right atrium is 75 percent with a $Po_2$ of 40 mm Hg. Blood returning from heart muscle via the coronary sinus has a saturation of only about 20 percent because of the large amount extracted by the heart muscle.

As mentioned earlier, the oxygen saturation of hemoglobin cannot exceed 100 percent. However, elevations in oxygen saturation of hemoglobin may occur relative to expected concentrations. The right heart chambers have normal saturations of 70 to 80 percent. A significant increase in these (venous) percentages indicates that oxygenated arterial blood is mixing with venous blood. A septal defect can produce this abnormality.

Reductions in the oxygen saturation indicate excessive extraction of oxygen by the tissue. Fever and acidosis are two conditions that reduce oxygen saturation, because they may result in excessive oxygen demand and, thus, excessive extraction of oxygen by tissue.

### Derived Hemodynamic Parameters

A number of other hemodynamic parameters can be derived from the direct parameters. These additional parameters are measures of cardiac contractility and afterload that are very helpful in determining the appropriate interventions. Derived hemodynamic parameters include stroke volume and stroke volume index, stroke work and stroke work index, systemic vascular resistance, pulmonary vascular resistance, coronary perfusion pressure, ejection fraction, and cardiac index. The normal ranges for these parameters are shown in Table 2–2.

Each of these derived parameters can be helpful in evaluating the contractility or functional capability of the heart. Cardiac function curves may be constructed from stroke work and pulmonary capillary wedge pressure measurements. Such curves differentiate the failing heart from the heart that is normal and from the heart that has increased contractility.

## Stroke Volume/Work

Stroke volume is the cardiac output divided by the heart rate, or the amount of blood ejected with each contraction. The normal stroke volume depends on the patient's size and level of activity. A normal range for stroke volume at rest is 60 to 130 ml/beat. The stroke volume index is obtained by dividing the stroke volume by the patient's body surface area. Like the cardiac index, this calculation adjusts the stroke volume for the patient's size. This parameter may be derived from echocardiograms, ventriculograms, and nuclear imaging (e.g., blood pool scans).

Another technique that is used to determine the functional capability of the heart is stroke work or stroke work index. Stroke work is the product of stroke volume and the pressure generated by the ventricle during contraction. The following formula can be used to determine stroke work:

**Table 2–2** Normal Ranges for Derived Hemodynamic Parameters

| Parameter | Acronym | Normal Range |
| --- | --- | --- |
| Cardiac output | CO | 4–8 liters/min |
| Cardiac index | CI | 2.5–4 liters/min |
| Stroke volume | SV | 60–130 ml/beat |
| Stroke volume index | SVI | 33–75 ml/beat/m² |
| Stroke work | SW | 45–85 g/beat (left ventricle) |
| Stroke work index | SWI | 66 ± 12 g/m² |
| Systemic vascular resistance | SVR | 800–1,600 dyne-seconds/cm$^{-5}$ |
| Pulmonary vascular resistance | PVR | 150–250 dyne-seconds/cm$^{-5}$ |
| Ejection fraction | EF | 65% ± 8% |
| Oxygen saturation | | |
|   Superior vena cava | | 70% |
|   Inferior vena cava | | 80% |
|   Right heart chamber | | 75% |
|   Pulmonary artery | | 75% |
|   Coronary sinus | | 20% |
|   Left heart chambers | | 96% |
| Arteriovenous oxygen | | |
|   difference | a-vDo₂ | 3–5.5 mg/dl |

$$SW = (MAP - EDP) \times SV \times 0.0136$$

where

$$
\begin{aligned}
SW &= \text{stroke work, measured in g/beat} \\
MAP &= \text{mean arterial pressure} \\
EDP &= \text{end-diastolic pressure of ventricle} \\
SV &= \text{stroke volume} \\
0.0136 &= \text{factor for conversion of pressure to work}
\end{aligned}
$$

This formula can be used to determine the stroke work of either ventricle by placing either the mean pulmonary arterial pressure or the mean systemic arterial pressure in the formula for $AP$. Once the stroke volume is known, this calculation can be done at the patient's bedside. The stroke work index is determined by dividing the stroke work by the body surface area. The stroke work index is expressed in $g/m^2$.

Hyperdynamic states that increase the stroke volume, such as exercise, also increase the stroke work index. Conditions that reduce the stroke volume result in a low stroke work index as well.

*Vascular Resistance*

The force that the ventricle must overcome to maintain blood flow, vascular resistance, can be used to determine ventricular work. Physiologically, this resistance increases as the arterioles constrict. Vascular resistance ($VR$) is equal to the difference ($\Delta$) in pressure divided by the cardiac output ($CO$). This number then must be converted to absolute units by means of a conversion factor of 80. The following formula can be adapted to measure systemic or pulmonary vascular resistance by substituting appropriate pressures:

$$VR = \frac{\Delta \text{ Pressure}}{CO} \times 80$$

Systemic vascular resistance ($SVR$) can be calculated as

$$SVR = \frac{MAP - RAP}{CO} \times 80$$

where $MAP$ is mean arterial pressure and $RAP$ is mean right atrial pressure. To adapt the formula for pulmonary vascular resistance ($PVR$), it is necessary to substitute only the pressure, as cardiac output and the conversion factor remain the same. The mean pulmonary artery pressure $(\overline{PAP})$ and mean pulmonary capillary wedge pressure ($\overline{PCWP}$) fit into the formula to determine pulmonary vascular resistance (*PVR*):

$$PVR = \frac{\overline{PAP} - \overline{PCWP}}{CO} \times 80$$

This calculation can be done at the patient's bedside without a computer.

Systemic and pulmonary vascular resistance are other measures of cardiac work. The resistance against which the ventricles pump (afterload) may be elevated or reduced. Reduced vascular resistance may be related to vasodilation, which may be physiologic or drug-induced. Vascular resistance is increased in the presence of vasoconstriction, a complex process that may be compensatory or pathological. Increased afterload may also result from various drugs (e.g., epinephrine, norepinephrine, dopamine).

*Coronary Perfusion Pressure*

Although not measured specifically, coronary perfusion pressure is an important parameter in hemodynamics. This is the amount of pressure required to perfuse the coronary circulation. Since the myocardium already extracts an extremely high percentage of oxygen from the blood, the supply of oxygen to the myocardium cannot be increased by increasing extraction, as is done with other tissue. The blood flow to the myocardium must be sustained, however, to prevent a decrease in the delivery of oxygenated blood and, consequently, a decrease in the oxygen supply to the myocardial tissue.

Because perfusion of the coronary circulation occurs primarily during diastole, the necessary pressure must be generated during diastole. Therefore, alterations in coronary perfusion pressure occur in relation to alterations in aortic diastolic pressure, and close attention to diastolic pressure is necessary to ensure adequate coronary perfusion. It is believed that optimal mean diastolic pressures are 60 to 80 mm Hg.

Coronary perfusion pressures may become too low with any drop in diastolic pressure. This may be associated with low circulating volumes. Because an adequate cardiac output is essential for adequate perfusion of the coronary vessels, a low cardiac output adversely affects coronary perfusion.

Increased coronary perfusion pressures result from increases in diastolic pressure. Vasoconstrictive drugs and increased vascular resistance for other reasons may be responsible for an elevated diastolic pressure. Intra-aortic balloon pumping increases coronary perfusion pressure by augmenting the diastolic pressure.

*Ejection Fraction*

Associated with stroke volume, the ejection fraction is the amount of blood ejected from the left ventricle with each contraction in relation to the total ventricular volume. Expressed as a percentage rather than a simple volume, the ejection fraction is yet another means for evaluating ventricular function. While a stroke volume of 70 ml/beat may be considered normal, it is much more satisfactory if that 70 ml is 70 percent of the total ventricular volume, rather than only 35 percent. An ejection fraction of less than 50 percent indicates serious ventricular dysfunction; less than 35 percent suggests dysfunction that is quite profound.

Ejection fractions may be determined by several means. During heart catheterization, a ventriculogram is usually performed, and this can be used to calculate an accurate ejection fraction. Nuclear imaging, such as blood pool scans, can also be used to determine the left ventricular ejection fraction accurately. Echocardiograms have been used to estimate stroke volume and chamber volume, but ejection fractions derived from these figures have been found to be somewhat inaccurate.

Those conditions that elevate the cardiac index also result in a high ejection fraction. High cardiac indexes or ejection fractions are of little concern, because they occur in heathy individuals. Similarly, ejection fractions are low in the same conditions in which the cardiac index is low. Such conditions as reduced ventricular compliance or contractility, excessive afterload, and abnormal preload produce low ejection fractions.

*Systolic Time Intervals*

Measurement of systolic time intervals may also be clinically useful. By simultaneously recording the ECG, phonocardiogram, and carotid pulse, the duration of the left ventricular preejection and ejection phases can be estimated. Normally, the ratio of left ventricular preejection to ejection time is 0.31 to 0.39. As the heart begins to fail, the ratio of the preejection to the ejection time increases, and ventricular filling time may be prolonged. Although changes in the ratio correlate well with other measurements of left ventricular function, this measurement does not indicate whether changes are related to preload or afterload, or whether they are related to contractility. Conduction and valvular abnormalities reduce the reliability of these measurements

*Cardiac Output/Index: The Fick Method*

The Fick method of cardiac output measurement is based on measurements of $Po_2$, $Pco_2$, and expired air; it is not usually done at the patient's bedside. This method is considered quite accurate and is used to test the accuracy of the other methods. The Fick method is based on the principles of Adolf Fick, who noted that oxygen uptake per unit of blood is reflected in the difference between the oxygen concentrations of arterial and mixed venous blood.[10]

In order to determine oxygen consumption, the oxygen removed from inspired air over a period of time is measured. If it is also possible to measure the oxygen concentration in arterial blood leaving the lungs and in mixed venous blood returning to the lungs, the amount of blood flowing through the lungs can be determined. With the Fick formula, these measurements can be used to calculate cardiac output ($CO$):

$$CO = \frac{O_2 \text{ consumption (ml/min)}}{\text{Arterial } O_2 \text{ content (mg/dl)} - \text{Venous } O_2 \text{ content (mg/dl)}}$$

Given these measurements,

$$
\begin{aligned}
O_2 \text{ consumption} &= 200 \text{ ml}\\
O_2 \text{ saturation (arterial)} &= 20 \text{ mg/dl}\\
O_2 \text{ saturation (mixed venous)} &= 12 \text{ mg/dl}
\end{aligned}
$$

the cardiac output ($CO$) can be calculated:

$$CO = \frac{200 \text{ ml/min}}{20 \text{ mg/dl} - 12 \text{ mg/dl}} = \frac{200 \text{ ml/min}}{8 \text{ mg/dl}} = \frac{200}{0.08} = 2{,}500 \text{ ml/min} = 2.5 \text{ liters/min}$$

Although the Fick method is quite accurate, it is difficult to obtain the measurements required.

The Fick method can also be used to estimate cardiac output. The steps in estimating the cardiac output are based on assumptions that may or may not be accurate, however; the less accurate the assumption, the less accurate the calculation. The steps used in an estimated calculation are as follows:[11]

1. Calculate the patient's body surface area (BSA) using the DuBois body surface chart.[12]
2. Multiply the BSA by the oxygen consumption per square meter. (In a basal metabolic state, this figure is 125 ml $O_2$ per m$^2$ BSA.)
3. Calculate the arteriovenous $O_2$ difference (a-vDo$_2$).
4. Divide the oxygen consumption by the calculated a-vDo$_2$.

The problems that surround this method arise from the many variations that occur. If the venous sample of blood used in the calculation is obtained from the central line in the superior vena cava, for instance, the oxygen level differs significantly from the oxygen level in a sample taken from the pulmonary artery, since the oxygen saturation of venous blood from the legs differs considerably from that of venous blood from the arms and head.

Individual variations in hemoglobin oxygen saturation can significantly alter calculations performed by the Fick method. Approximately 99 percent of the oxygen carried in the blood is bound to hemoglobin in a loose, reversible bond. Because of the rapid exchange that occurs in the lungs, the saturation of hemoglobin with oxygen nears 100 percent even when the heart rate is rapid; because of the mixture of unoxygenated blood from the bronchial circulation, the saturation of hemoglobin moving into the arterial circulation is reduced to 95 to 97 percent. When the highly saturated hemoglobin reaches the tissues, the oxygen is released for cellular use, and the saturation is reduced to approximately 75 percent as the blood returns to the heart.[13] Such variations can alter assumptions about resting oxygen consumption.

The arteriovenous oxygen difference is the difference between the oxygen saturation of arterial blood and the oxygen saturation of venous blood. If the difference is less than normal, less oxygen than normal has been extracted by the tissues, or a left-to-right cardiac shunt has contributed oxygenated blood to the mixed venous sample. A difference greater than normal suggests that there is a problem with oxygenation of the blood (e.g., pulmonary ventilation or diffusion problems) or that cardiac output is low, slowing circulation and allowing the tissues more time for extraction of oxygen.

The cardiac output or index is a major determinant of interventions in caring for cardiac patients. The cardiac index is more specific in that it accounts for patient size. An increased cardiac index is a normal response to specific physiologic states. Exercise and mild tachyarrhythmias, for example, may elevate the cardiac index in a healthy heart.

The cardiac index may decrease as a result of preload abnormalities, decreased contractility, excessive afterload, or abnormal heart rate or rhythms. Preload abnormalities can result in a decreased cardiac output. If the blood volume returning to the left ventricle is low, the stroke volume and, therefore, the cardiac index is reduced. On the other hand, excessive preload may stretch the myocardium beyond the optimum point on the cardiac function curve (see Figure 1–16), resulting in a decrease in the cardiac index.

A reduction in the cardiac index may result from decreased myocardial contractility caused by infarction, heart failure, constrictive disease, or cardiomyopathies. Ischemia of the myocardium and electrolyte imbalances that affect the movement of calcium may also reduce contractility, stroke volume, and the cardiac index.

When the heart must pump against an excessive afterload, its work increases, potentially decreasing contractility, stroke volume, and the cardiac index. Valvular stenosis and hypertension may cause such an excessive afterload.

Tachyarrhythmias and irregular cardiac rhythms may interfere with ventricular filling through reduced filling time, loss of atrioventricular synchrony, or loss of atrial kick. These conditions reduce stroke volume or interfere with systolic ejection. The result may be a reduction in cardiac output.

## INTERRELATIONSHIPS IN HEMODYNAMIC ALTERATIONS

Changes in a number of hemodynamic variables may affect the cardiac output and the numerous cardiovascular pressures. The body's ability to compensate for the changes can further complicate the complex activities of cardiopulmonary function.

### General Cardiovascular Causes of Changes in Hemodynamic Parameters

*Heart Rate and Rhythm*

With regular rhythms, the normal heart rate of 60 to 100 beats/min maintains an adequate cardiac output if all other factors are normal. The body may compensate for abnormalities in contractility, preload, and afterload by changing the heart rate, however. An increase in heart rate not only increases contractility and ventricular wall tension,[14] but also causes a more rapid rise of intraventricular pressure. This in turn reduces the duration of the ejection phase. Diastole may then be more prolonged, and coronary blood flow and ventricular filling may improve.

Even if an increase in heart rate has no effect on contractility, it increases cardiac output to some degree. If stroke volume is constant, an increased heart rate increases cardiac output. As the heart rate becomes excessively high, however, the diastolic filling time is reduced, which then reduces stroke volume and cardiac output.

Reductions in heart rate below normal levels decrease cardiac output, if all other factors remain constant. In very few situations are the other factors constant, however. Reductions in heart rate prolong the diastolic filling time to some degree, allowing more blood to enter the ventricle; this increases the stretch and preload of the myocardium. With the increased stretch come increased intracardiac pressures and contractility to compensate for the slower rate. Unfortunately, as bradycardias become very pronounced (i.e., 20 to 40 beats/min), the heart is unable to compensate fully, cardiac performance is impaired, and a reduction in cardiac output results.

Irregular heart rhythms or dysrhythmias affect intracardiac pressures and cardiac output in a number of ways. Atrial dysrhythmias are significant primarily in their effect on ventricular filling time or atrial systole. Premature atrial contractions reduce significantly the ventricular filling time. This adversely affects cardiac output, especially if such premature contractions are frequent. Atrial tachycardia has such a high rate (i.e., 160 to 220 beats/min) that the reduced ventricular filling time associated with it reduces cardiac output. Healthy hearts may or may not be able to compensate for this, but the severity of decreased cardiac output symptoms usually correlates with the extent of pathological cardiac disease.

Atrial flutter may compromise cardiac output through a reduction in ventricular filling time or through the loss of atrial kick (atrial systole) and, thus, the loss of that contribution to cardiac output. Hemodynamic decompensation as a result of rapid ventricular response to atrial flutter may have dire consequences and certainly has a significant effect on cardiac output, especially in a patient with cardiac disease. Because atrial fibrillation eliminates the atrial contribution to ventricular filling, it adversely affects cardiac output. The fibrillating atria disrupt normal hemodynamics and may result in stasis of blood in the atria, which can lead to fatal clot formation.

Junctional dysrhythmias may disrupt cardiac hemodynamics by one of several mechanisms. Alterations in the normal atrium-to-ventricle sequence may adversely affect ventricular filling, reducing cardiac output. Like bradycardias, slow junctional rhythms may also reduce cardiac output; furthermore, they disrupt the normal sequence of cardiac events. Junctional tachycardias with rates as high as 250 beats/min may compromise cardiac output through their effect on ventricular filling.

Second- and third-degree heart blocks may result in a reduced cardiac output. The slow heart rates associated with heart blocks and the effect of the disruption of the cardiac cycle on ventricular filling may be causative factors.

Ventricular dysrhythmias also reduce cardiac output. Premature ventricular contractions and ventricular tachycardia, for example, reduce cardiac output by reducing ventricular filling time. Ventricular tachycardia also disrupts the atrioventricular sequence of contraction, decreasing cardiac output even more. Ventricular tachycardia may deteriorate into ventricular fibrillation, in which there is no cardiac output. Although the ventricular escape rhythm does not generally provide adequate cardiac output, it may be temporarily life-saving with third-degree heart block.

*Circulating Blood Volume*

Alterations in circulating blood volume affect the intracardiac pressures and the cardiac output. Any increase in blood volume tends to increase venous return to the heart, resulting in an increase in CVP and in cardiac output. Increases in venous return usually increase preload, with greater contractility contributing to an improved cardiac output. In a patient whose heart is failing, however, an increase in the circulating volume and venous return may reduce contractility and cardiac output. Although a sudden increase in the circulating blood volume may even double the cardiac output, it gradually returns to normal as the veins distend to reduce venous return and as shunting from the capillaries to the tissues occurs.

Circulating blood volume may be reduced through any one of several mechanisms, including hemorrhage, extravascular shunting, and renal excretion because of disease or drugs. Such mechanisms as decreases in pressure and increases in heart rates compensate for reductions in circulating volume to some extent. Significant reductions in circulating volume, however, result in a significant drop in cardiac output.

*Myocardial Contractility*

There is a direct relationship between myocardial contractility and cardiac output. The force of myocardial contraction may increase as a result of changes in several factors (e.g., preload, afterload, and heart rate), and it may be affected by hypoxemia, electrolyte cardiac disease, or sympathetic nerve activity. As contractility increases in response to changes in calcium flow, heart rate, increased preload, and/or release of cathecholamines by the sympathetic nervous system, cardiac output increases. Intracardiac pressures may rise as a result of increased contractility. Hypoxemia secondary to inadequate coronary perfusion, alterations in calcium flow secondary to electrolyte disturbances, and cardiac disease may adversely affect contractility, reducing intracardiac pressures and cardiac output.

*Vascular Distensibility*

The ability of vessels to distend is an important compensatory mechanism that helps to prevent cardiac failure when the circulating blood volume has increased. Distensibility of veins provides a significant capacitance in those vessels, while distensibility of arteries provides only limited capacitance. Venodilation reduces the mean circulatory pressure and, thus, cardiac output.

Changes in the vasomotor tone of the arterioles does not significantly affect the mean circulatory pressure or the distribution of total blood volume. Because of the afterload reduction that occurs with vasodilation, cardiac output increases. Vasoconstriction increases the afterload, requiring more cardiac work and reducing cardiac output.

## Noncardiac Contributions to Hemodynamic Alterations

Other body systems play an important role in alterations of hemodynamic parameters. These alterations, which range from compensatory to pathological, may be simple or complex.

*Pulmonary Contribution*

Variations in hemodynamic parameters that involve the pulmonary system are related primarily to two of the processes of pulmonary function and gas exchange:

(1) ventilation, defined as the movement of air in and out of the lungs, and (2) diffusion, defined as the movement of gases back and forth among the alveoli, the plasma, and red blood cells.

The body has several mechanisms to deliver the amount of oxygen required by the various tissues. An increase in ventilation is one such mechanism. Increases in the depth and rate of ventilation occur in response to chemical or neurologic stimuli. A low $Pao_2$, low pH, and a high $Paco_2$, all conditions that may result from inadequate ventilation or abnormal diffusion, stimulate chemoreceptors located in the aortic arch and carotid sinus. Stimulation of these chemoreceptors results in an increased respiratory rate and vasoconstriction of resistance vessels. This vasoconstriction increases afterload and intracardiac pressures, as well as cardiac work.

The heart rate may or may not increase with the stimulation of chemoreceptors, depending on the patient's ventilatory status. If the respiratory rate increases, but is not controlled, the heart rate increases because of hypocapnia and because of the excessive movements associated with the increase in ventilation. Control of ventilation and the respiratory rate (mechanically or with drugs) during stimulation of chemoreceptors results in bradycardia, various degrees of atrioventricular heart block, and a reduction of left ventricular contractility.

The left ventricle's response to ventilation and diffusion is biphasic. Hypoxemia initially stimulates chemoreceptors and causes a transient depression of contractility of the left ventricle. This depression reduces arterial and intracardiac pressures, as well as cardiac output. The body then compensates for these decreases through a mechanism called the central nervous system ischemic response, which elevates arterial blood pressure through vasoconstriction. This elevated pressure increases blood flow and, by increasing left ventricular contractility, increases the cardiac output; this is the body's attempt to restore normal cardiac output. Severe hypoxemia depresses myocardial contractility despite compensatory responses, since the cardiac muscle requires sufficient oxygen to function.

*Renal Contribution*

The role of the renal system in hemodynamics is very complex. The renal system controls fluid balance through excretion or retention of electrolytes and water. Through fluid manipulation, the renal system helps to control arterial pressure and, therefore, hemodynamics.

Excretion of sodium and water directly reduces circulating blood volume, thus reducing arterial blood pressure. Conversely, when a reduction in the circulating blood volume results in a drop in arterial pressure, the renal system takes a series of actions to conserve water. The actions involve yet another body system—the autonomic nervous system.

*Autonomic Nervous System*

When there is a reduction in the circulating volume, the sympathetic nervous system releases epinephrine and norepinephrine (catecholamines), both of which reduce renal blood flow and stimulate the release of renin to initiate the renin-angiotensin system. This mechanism effects the release of aldosterone and an increase in antidiuretic hormone. These hormones regulate the excretion and reabsorption of sodium and water to increase extracellular fluid volume, cardiac output, and blood pressure.

The release of epinephrine and norepinephrine may be a response to a variety of stimuli, including exercise and stress, as well as to reduced blood pressure and cardiac output. The release of these hormones from the adrenal medulla is controlled by the sympathetic nervous system. In addition to the changes that they produce in blood pressure, these hormones increase the heart rate.

Stimulation of the parasympathetic nervous system has an effect opposite to that of stimulation of the sympathetic nervous system. The parasympathetic actions influence predominantly the sinoatrial node and, therefore, the heart rate. These two nervous systems are coordinated through the baroreceptors located in the aortic arch and carotid sinus. If blood pressure rises suddenly, these stretch receptors send impulses to the medulla, which then inhibits vasoconstriction (sympathetic activity) and causes peripheral vasodilation. The impulses also stimulate the vagal center, reducing myocardial contractility (parasympathetic activity) and producing bradycardia. The converse is true if the pressure drops—there is decreased stretch, reduced stimulation of the parasympathetic center, and reduced inhibition of the sympathetic center.

## CLINICAL APPLICATION

Critical illnesses of several types alter hemodynamic parameters. Obviously, it is essential to understand the principles related to the various parameters and to apply the data obtained from monitoring the hemodynamics to the clinical situation.

### Cardiac Failure

Simply defined, cardiac failure refers to the heart's inability to pump enough blood to meet the tissue demands. When cardiac failure occurs, the sympathetic nervous system normally responds with a number of acute compensatory mechanisms to restore normal blood flow. The specific alterations in hemodynamic parameters that occur with cardiac failure depend on the severity of the failure. The compensatory responses often further complicate the hemodynamic picture.

The CVP may be normal or elevated. If the heart failure is primarily left-sided, the CVP is initially normal. If the heart failure progresses to the right side or if it is originally right-sided, the CVP is elevated. Inability of the right ventricle to pump adequately (e.g., because of elevated preload, reduced contractility, or elevated afterload) may be responsible for the elevated CVP.

Arterial pressures may be elevated, normal, or low. Measurement of these pressures is of limited usefulness in determining the cardiopulmonary status of a patient. It may be useful to monitor the arterial pressure for changes, however; such data, in combination with other data, may be helpful in the assessment of the patient's clinical status.

The pulmonary capillary wedge pressure is probably the most helpful parameter in determining the clinical status of the patient with cardiac failure. An excellent parameter for determining left ventricular function, the pulmonary capillary wedge pressure can be obtained rather simply by use of a Swan-Ganz catheter. A rapid elevation in this pressure, especially to a level greater than 20 to 25 mm Hg, signifies severe left ventricular failure.

As the pulmonary capillary wedge pressure indirectly reflects left ventricular pressure, this pressure is also elevated with cardiac failure. Right ventricular pressures, such as the CVP, may be elevated if the right ventricle has failed.

Early or mild cardiac failure does not produce a significant reduction in the cardiac output/index. As the ventricle becomes increasingly less capable of pumping enough blood to meet tissue oxygen demands, however, the cardiac output begins to fall. Measurement of cardiac output provides the information necessary to determine the cardiac function curve and several derived hemo-dynamic parameters. This information can be used in planning interventions.

As the cardiac output falls, alterations in the extraction of oxygen by tissues may change the hemoglobin oxygen saturation. More oxygen is extracted in low output states, resulting in lower mixed venous saturations. Unless the pulmonary congestion often associated with left ventricular failure reduces the oxygen/carbon dioxide diffusion, the arterial oxygen saturation may be normal. The a-vDo$_2$ may be greater, however, because more oxygen has been extracted.

Systemic vascular resistance is usually unchanged at first. Changes may be noted, however, as compensatory responses (e.g., vasoconstriction) occur via the sympathetic nervous system. The pulmonary vascular resistance may be elevated or normal, depending on the cause of the cardiac failure. If the cardiac failure is related to pulmonary disease, the pulmonary vascular resistance may be elevated.

As discussed earlier, stroke volume and stroke work are related to cardiac output. When cardiac output decreases, stroke volume and stroke work, as well as their respective indexes, decrease. This may be at least temporarily countered by the compensatory action of the body.

Owing to the inadequate pumping function of the myocardium, the ejection function in cardiac failure is generally reduced below normal. It is difficult to assess coronary perfusion pressure, but changes in myocardial perfusion are clearly related to cardiac output; therefore, when reductions in cardiac output occur, myocardial perfusion may be jeopardized.

Interventions used in the treatment of heart failure may be specifically related to the alterations in hemodynamic parameters. Because heart failure may be associated with increased preload, reduced contractility, and/or increased afterload, such interventions are based on these factors. For example, intervention for an increased preload may include reduction in venous return through diuresis, vasodilation, or patient positioning. This intervention may reduce the CVP and the pulmonary capillary wedge pressure as well.

The administration of vasodilating drugs to reduce cardiac work by reducing vascular resistance is common in the management of cardiac failure. In addition, this intervention may assist in reducing preload by reducing venous return through venodilation of capacitance vessels.

It is also important to improve contractility in the failing heart. Serial measurements of cardiac output help to determine the progress. Inotropic drugs, such as dopamine, dobutamine, and digitalis, are good choices to achieve this goal.

Continuous monitoring of the hemodynamic parameters discussed is important not only to identify the onset or progression of cardiac failure, but also to determine the effectiveness of treatment.

## Shock

It is possible to classify shock in several different ways. Hemodynamic parameters may be used both to help differentiate the types of shock and to determine which interventions are appropriate. In general, shock may be considered a severe pathophysiologic syndrome that causes an abnormality in cellular metabolism. The three major types of shock are hypovolemic, cardiogenic, and septic shock (Table 2–3).

Early diagnosis of shock is important so that the process can be reversed before deterioration of vital organs has become extensive. The general hemodynamic changes that occur with shock include

- a reduction in blood pressure with an associated reduction in urine output
- a rapid heart rate
- cold and clammy skin
- metabolic acidosis

Blood pressure components include systolic, diastolic, and pulse pressure. Systolic pressure is determined by a combination of such factors as stroke volume and

**Table 2–3** Early Differentiation of Shock: Changes in Parameters

|  | Hypovolemic | Cardiogenic | Septic |
|---|---|---|---|
| Systolic blood pressure | No change | No change or ↓ | No change or ↓ |
| Diastolic blood pressure | ↑ | ↑ | ↑ or no change |
| Pulse pressure | ↓ | ↓ | ↓ |
| Stroke volume | ↓ | ↓ | ↓↑ or no change |
| Cardiac output | ↓ | No change or ↓ | ↑↓ |
| Heart rate | ↑ | ↑↓ | ↑ or no change |
| Peripheral vascular resistance | ↑ | ↑ | ↑ or no change |
| Pulmonary capillary wedge pressure | ↓ | ↑ | ↓ or no change |
| Stroke work | ↓ | ↓ | ↓ or no change |
| Central venous pressure | ↓ | No change or ↓↑ | ↑↓ or no change |

afterload. Diastolic pressure correlates with the amount of vasoconstriction. Pulse pressure is associated with stroke volume and aortic rigidity.

In hypovolemic shock, stroke volume and pulse pressure decrease long before the pressure falls. As the sympathetic nervous system responds to the fall in stroke volume, causing vasoconstriction, diastolic pressure rises. The systolic pressure can usually be maintained for some time. Associated with the low stroke volume and low pulse pressure is a low cardiac output, which frequently can be noted before the fall in systolic pressure that has historically been the key sign of shock. The pulmonary capillary wedge pressure and stroke work are also below normal in hypovolemic shock. Increased peripheral vascular resistance and an increased heart rate are compensatory mechanisms that are symptomatic of hypovolemic shock. Because of these compensatory mechanisms, cardiac output may be normal or even high.

Cardiogenic shock is very similar to hypovolemic shock in a number of ways. In cardiogenic shock, the problem is not a lack of volume, but rather the heart's inability to pump that volume. Most cardiogenic shock patients have a reduced stroke volume, reduced cardiac output, increased heart rate, and increased peripheral vascular resistance. Some patients may also have slow heart rates related to ischemia of the inferior left ventricle.

Shock related to severe sepsis is one of the most difficult types of shock to diagnose, because it may be hypodynamic or hyperdynamic. Hypodynamic septic shock creates a relative or absolute hypovolemia because of capillary leakage. Hyperdynamic septic shock prevents normal cell metabolism and may produce shunting and an abnormal distribution of blood flow. Because of these opposite states, the blood pressure may be decreased or unchanged, and the cardiac output may be increased or decreased. The stroke volume may decrease, increase, or remain unchanged. Close observation of the patient who may have sepsis is essential.

Monitoring of these patients should include—but not be limited to—blood pressure, heart rate and rhythm, respirations, pulmonary capillary wedge pressure, and CVP. Graphing the changes in these parameters is helpful in early intervention.

Treatment of shock may be extremely detrimental if the diagnosis is not precise. Therefore, it is essential that parameters be observed carefully. If the patient has a volume deficit, for example, fluid therapy is necessary; an elevated pulmonary capillary wedge pressure indicates a need to reduce circulating volume, however. Increased peripheral vascular resistance (afterload) may indicate the need for vasodilation. If the patient has a low systolic pressure, low cardiac output, reduced coronary perfusion, and high afterload, it may be necessary to use the intra-aortic balloon pump to improve cardiac output and coronary perfusion, while reducing afterload and, therefore, cardiac work.

**Cardiac Tamponade**

Diagnosis of cardiac tamponade is a challenge. As little as 100 ml blood, if accumulating rapidly, may produce tamponade. Hemodynamic parameters change at varying rates, depending on the speed with which tamponade occurs. The alterations occur in response to physiologic changes in the pericardial sac.

Generally, the CVP is elevated as a result of the ventricle's inability to stretch and fill during diastole, which prevents venous return. This rise in venous pressure alters the waveforms of the venous pressure. Both a and v waves are usually prominent with rapid x and y descents. As diastolic filling is reduced, the stroke volume and pulse pressure also fall. The systolic blood pressure falls, and tachycardia develops to compensate for a low cardiac output.

Of special hemodynamic significance in patients with cardiac tamponade is the presence of pulsus paradoxus. Defined as a decline of 10 mm Hg or more in the systolic blood pressure during normal inspiration, pulsus paradoxus is detected by checking cuff blood pressure during inspiration and expiration. If the difference between the systolic pressure heard during expiration only and the systolic pressure heard equally well during both inspiration and expiration is greater than

10 mm Hg, cardiac compression is present. Kussmaul's sign, which is a rise rather than the physiologic fall in venous pressure with inspiration, is usually present in patients with cardiac tamponade.

Cardiac tamponade must be differentiated from constrictive pericarditis. While measures of hemodynamic parameters may be similar in both disorders, constrictive pericarditis is a chronic condition that occurs over a longer period of time. Symptoms of right ventricular failure accompany the condition. Pulmonary and systemic venous pressures become equal over time, and pulsus paradoxus is less common.

Treatment of cardiac tamponade is designed to relieve the pressure on the heart and to remove the cause. Evacuation of the fluid in the pericardium via pericardiocentesis is usually necessary to reverse the abnormal hemodynamic parameters. Although complications may occur, this procedure generally restores the CVP to normal; stroke volume, blood pressure, and cardiac output rise to normal as well. Heart rate then falls in response to the other changes.

### Hypertension

Defined as a chronic elevation of the arterial blood pressure, hypertension has varied causes, including renal disease, vascular disorders, endocrine malfunctions, brain lesions, and drugs. Hypertension may also be related to none of these (i.e., essential hypertension). The associated abnormal hemodynamic parameters are not limited to the blood pressure.

As blood pressure rises, the afterload or resistance against which the heart pumps is increased, and systemic vascular resistance is elevated. The stroke volume may or may not be affected. The normal heart overcomes the elevated afterload by increasing contractility and heart rate as necessary. Initially, cardiac output is usually normal or elevated. As hypertension becomes more severe, cardiac output may drop in relation to the increased cardiac work and inability of the heart to pump adequately (heart failure).

Several treatments are available to eliminate the cause of hypertension and reduce the blood pressure. The success of therapy is measured by the change in blood pressure. Interventions include dietary restriction of salt to reduce circulating volume through renal excretion of water, weight loss, and stress reduction.

Medications are often prescribed for patients with hypertension. Diuretics are first-line drugs to reduce circulatory volume. Inhibitors that reduce sympathetic outflow from the brain reduce blood pressure. Finally, vasodilators relax vascular smooth muscle in the arterioles. All the antihypertensive medications have side-effects that may produce more problems than does hypertension, however.

---

**NOTES**

1. Nancy Meyer Holloway, *Nursing the Critically Ill Adult*, 2nd ed. (Menlo Park, Calif.: Addison-Wesley, 1984), 110–111.

2.  George P. Haag, "Central Venous Catheters and Monitoring," *Critical Care Quarterly* 2 (September 1979):51–55.

3.  Cathie E. Guzetta and Barbara Montgomery Dossey, *Cardiovascular Nursing Bodymind Tapestry* (St. Louis: C.V. Mosby, 1984), 113–114.

4.  American Edwards Laboratories, *Understanding Hemodynamic Measurements Made with the Swan-Ganz Catheter* (Santa Ana, Calif.: American Edwards Laboratories, 1982), 21.

5.  Elaine Keiss Daily and John Speer Schroeder, *Techniques in Bedside Hemodynamic Monitoring*, 2nd ed. (St. Louis: C.V. Mosby, 1981), 67.

6.  Jeanne L. Laulive, "Pulmonary Artery Pressures and Position Changes in the Critically Ill Adult," *Dimensions of Critical Care Nursing* 1:1 (1982): 28–34.

7.  American Edwards Laboratories, *Understanding Hemodynamic Measurements*, 16–17.

8.  Ibid., 18–19.

9.  Eugene F. DuBois, *Basal Metabolism in Health and Disease* (Philadelphia: Lea & Febiger, 1936).

10.  Daily and Schroeder, *Bedside Hemodynamic Monitoring*, 114.

11.  Ibid., 115.

12.  DuBois, *Basal Metabolism*, 1936.

13.  Carol Porth, *Pathophysiology: Concepts of Altered Health States* (Philadelphia: J.B. Lippincott, 1982), 262.

14.  Guzetta and Dossey, *Cardiovascular Nursing*, 518.

# Part II

# Case Studies

# Chapter 3

# Multiple Trauma

*Judy Dixon Fox, R.N., M.S.N.*

The number of people treated in hospitals for traumatic injuries each year has been growing steadily. Moreover, there has been an increase in the severity and complexity of those injuries.[1] The management of trauma patients can be very challenging to all members of the health care team, partly because of the unpredictable nature of traumatic injuries. There are, however, many physiologic changes that occur in all severely injured patients, regardless of the extent of injury. Many of these physiologic changes directly or indirectly affect hemodynamic homeostasis. Such physiologic alterations include hypovolemia, hypermetabolic state, and altered oxygen transport.[2-5]

> Mr. H was a 22-year-old man involved in a motor vehicle accident. Having sustained multiple system injuries, he was brought to the emergency department (ED).

## HEMODYNAMIC MONITORING FOR THE TRAUMA PATIENT

Severely injured patients have usually lost blood from either external or internal bleeding sites. The blood loss results in varying degrees of hypovolemia, which can change many hemodynamic parameters. Volume deficits may be reflected by decreases in cardiac filling pressures, such as right atrial and pulmonary capillary wedge pressures. If compensation mechanisms for the hypovolemia are inadequate, the low filling pressures result in a decreased cardiac output, cardiac index, and mean arterial pressure. The degree to which pressures change depends on the amount of volume loss, as well as on the ability of the individual to compensate for that loss.[6-9]

The body's attempts to compensate for hypovolemia and maintain an adequate mean arterial pressure lead to changes in those factors that determine cardiac output, including increases in heart rate, myocardial contractile force, and peripheral vasoconstriction. A reflection of afterload, vasoconstriction occurs in an attempt to shift volume to the core circulation and, thus, increase filling pressures; it can be monitored by using the derived parameter of systemic vascular resistance. If hypovolemia is not corrected or loss of volume continues, changes occur in both the direct and derived parameters. Therefore, mean arterial pressure, cardiac output, cardiac index, pulmonary capillary wedge pressure, and systemic vascular resistance can be used as indicators and monitors of shock states.[10–12]

Hypermetabolism increases cellular energy production and oxygen consumption. The increased cellular activity provides the energy necessary for compensations, wound healing, and immune responses. Although the hypermetabolic rate can be maintained for several days, it may be insufficient for the body's needs. If the body's oxygen and metabolic demands are not met, shock states may occur; the cardiac output, cardiac index, and mean arterial pressure decreases, and the systemic vascular resistance increases.[13–16]

Alteration in oxygen transport is often a problem following severe trauma. Not only does the decreased perfusion pressure associated with hypovolemia make it difficult to transport available oxygen to the various tissues and organs, but also the blood's ability to carry the oxygen may be affected. Because oxygen is transported by hemoglobin, low hemoglobin levels secondary to loss of blood volume result in poor oxygen-carrying capacity. As the available oxygen becomes inadequate to meet cellular demands, hypoxia develops. Changes within the pulmonary vasculature that are produced by hypoxia can be monitored by means of the derived parameter of pulmonary vascular resistance.[17,18]

> On arrival at the ED, Mr. H was responsive to verbal stimulus. His skin was pale, cool, and diaphoretic. There were numerous abrasions on his extremities and areas of ecchymoses around his hips, left thigh, and buttocks. His abdomen was distended and firm. He had been receiving 40 percent oxygen ($O_2$) via mask during transport, and this was continued in the ED. Initial blood pressure was 70/40 mm Hg, with a mean arterial pressure of 51 mm Hg and a respiratory rate of 44/min. The cardiac monitor showed sinus tachycardia of 139/min. A peritoneal lavage showed the presence of blood, and a serum hematocrit was reported as 27 percent, indicative of intra-abdominal bleeding. Radiographic examination revealed fractures of the pelvis and left femur.
>
> A central venous line was inserted into Mr. H's left internal jugular vein. The opening central venous pressure (CVP) was recorded as 1 cm $H_2O$. Ringer's lactate solution had been infused peripherally at a wide open rate during transport to the ED, and the infusion was continued through the central line. A dopamine drip was initiated and antishock pants applied on admission to the ED. These procedures, along with the

continual infusion of fluids and blood, as it became available, brought the CVP to 3 cm $H_2O$, blood pressure to 88/64 mm Hg, and mean arterial pressure to 72 mm Hg. A Foley catheter had been inserted to monitor urine output closely. Measures to stabilize Mr. H's condition were continued until he was taken to surgery.

## MANAGEMENT OF HEMODYNAMIC VARIABLES

Often, the most dramatic shock states are seen in the ED. During this early period, several hemodynamic changes occur, but many of the alterations are not measurable without the use of sophisticated pressure monitoring devices. In Mr. H's case, the pulmonary artery catheter was not inserted until he reached the operating room. The patient's hypovolemic state could still be determined from the limited parameters available, however. The low CVP reflected a decreased right atrial filling pressure, while the hypotension reflected a low cardiac output. Physiologic compensations to accommodate these low pressures were evidenced by several physical findings. For example, a marked sinus tachycardia was present, indicating the body's attempt to increase stroke volume and cardiac output. Although there was no way to calculate systemic and pulmonary vascular resistance, cool skin and pallor indicated peripheral vasoconstriction. Blood gas levels were used to determine oxygen transport.

The administration of fluids was not enough to replace the volume losses that resulted from Mr. H's injuries. Adjunctive measures to assist the patient's own compensatory mechanisms included the application of antishock pants and the dopamine drip. Antishock pants are designed to assist with plasma expansion through the mechanism of volume displacement. The abdominal compartment and each leg compartment can be inflated at different pressures to increase the systemic vascular resistance and displace volume from the lower extremities and peritoneum into the core circulation. The effectiveness of antishock pants in the management of hypovolemia has long been established, but its mechanism of action in improving the mean arterial pressure and cardiac output is still under investigation. In the past, it was believed that inflation of the antishock pants displaced large amounts of blood from the lower extremities. More recent research findings indicate that the actual volume displacement may be little more than 500 ml and that the primary action of the antishock pants is through the manipulation of the systemic vascular resistance.[19,20] Dopamine also increases the systemic vascular resistance and, through its inotropic properties, can increase the myocardial contractile force to improve stroke volume.[21,22] The effectiveness of these adjuncts were evidenced by Mr. H in increases in CVP, blood pressure, and mean arterial pressure.

Mr. H underwent a splenectomy and had a liver laceration surgically repaired. The fractured femur was placed in skeletal traction; the pelvic fracture did not require internal fixation. After surgery, the patient was admitted to the intensive care unit (ICU) with numerous invasive lines in place. Two large-bore peripheral intravenous (IV) lines and the left internal jugular line were used for the transfusion of blood and fresh-frozen plasma. A pulmonary artery catheter with an extra infusion port had been inserted into the right subclavian artery, and both the right atrial and extra infusion port were used to infuse Ringer's lactate solution.

The selection of fluids and the management of volume replacement have been topics of much clinical research. Data support the use of colloid solutions combined with crystalloids in the management of hypovolemic shock, and many comparative studies have been done on the effectiveness of various colloid and crystalloid solutions, including artificial preparations. Because of its close resemblance to extracellular fluid, Ringer's lactate solution continues to be the crystalloid of choice for rapid volume replacement. Hetastarch (Hespan) is an artificial colloid solution now being used in the treatment of hypovolemia. Its relatively low cost has been cited as one of its advantages. Furthermore, Hespan has not been associated with the coagulopathy that caused practitioners to cease using Dextran in fluid resuscitation. Clinical research continues over appropriate choices and combinations of solutions in the treatment of hypovolemic shock.[23,24]

On admission to the ICU, Mr. H was responsive, but very sedated. He had two abdominal drains and a nasogastric tube in place. A radial artery line had been inserted for continuous monitoring of systolic, diastolic, and mean arterial pressures. The pulmonary artery line was connected to a transducer for monitoring of pulmonary artery and pulmonary capillary wedge pressures. The IV infusion rate of crystalloid solutions totaled 250 ml/hour. Mr. H was maintaining a mean arterial pressure of 65 to 75 mm Hg without the use of dopamine or antishock pants. Urine output was good. The 40 percent $O_2$ mask remained in place, although blood gas values in the recovery room were good. A postoperative hematocrit was reported as 29.4 percent. The monitor showed a sinus tachycardia, and pressure waveforms from the radial and pulmonary artery catheters were normal. Soon after arrival into the ICU, a complete hemodynamic evaluation was done (Table 3–1).

As the infusion of fluid and blood products continued, positive changes were noted in Mr. H's blood pressure, mean arterial pressure, pulmonary artery pressure, and pulmonary capillary wedge pressure. Fresh-frozen plasma and whole blood were transfused to replace cellular

**Table 3–1** Hemodynamic Profile

| Parameter | Time of Admission to the ICU | 12 Hours after Admission | Postoperative Day 4 |
|---|---|---|---|
| Blood pressure | 108/52 mm Hg | 118/70 mm Hg | 132/80 mm Hg |
| Heart rate | 132/min | 110/min | 88/min |
| Respiration rate | 22/min | 24/min | 22/min |
| Temperature | 98° F | 98.8°F | 98.6°F |
| Pulmonary artery pressure | 22/9 mm Hg | 24/10 mm Hg | 26/14 mm Hg |
| Pulmonary capillary wedge pressure | 6 mm Hg | 8 mm Hg | 10 mm Hg |
| Mean arterial pressure | 70 mm Hg | 86 mm Hg | 97 mm Hg |
| Right atrial pressure | 5 mm Hg | 6 mm Hg | 11 mm Hg |
| Cardiac output | 3.5 liters/min | 4.8 liters/min | 6.52 liters/min |
| Cardiac index | 2.03 liters/min/m² | 2.79 liters/min/m² | 3.79 liters/min/m² |
| Pulmonary vascular resistance | 160 dyne-sec/cm$^{-5}$ | 117 dyne-sec/cm$^{-5}$ | 183 dyne-sec/cm$^{-5}$ |
| Systemic vascular resistance | 1,485 dyne-sec/cm$^{-5}$ | 1,333 dyne-sec/cm$^{-5}$ | 1,055 dyne-sec/cm$^{-5}$ |

components and clotting factors lost through hemorrhage. Within 8 hours after admission to the ICU, Mr. H had received 2,000 ml fluid, 4 units fresh-frozen plasma, and 3 units whole blood. The hematocrit was 34 percent, and blood pressure was stable with a mean arterial pressure of 85 to 90 mm Hg and a pulmonary artery end-diastolic pressure of 8 to 9 mm Hg. At this time, the IV fluids were decreased to a total of 175 ml/hour and changed from Ringer's lactate solution to 5% dextrose, 45% normal saline (D5½NS). The monitor showed a sinus tachycardia of 114/min. Stabilization and improvement of parameters indicated effective management of the patient's hypovolemia. Effectiveness was further evidenced by another hemodynamic profile done 12 hours after admission to the ICU (see Table 3–1).

After the 12-hour hemodynamic profile had been obtained, IV fluids were decreased to a total of 125 ml/hour, and one of the two peripheral IV lines was discontinued. Mr. H was awake, alert, and oriented. His skin was warm and dry. There were no bowel sounds, and Mr. H remained on nasogastric suction, receiving nothing by mouth.

Mr. H progressed without adverse complications. On postoperative day 1, the administration of oxygen was discontinued. Hematocrit was 36 percent; mean arterial pressure was 90 to 95 mm Hg. On postoperative day 2, the arterial line was discontinued. The pulmonary artery catheter was discontinued on postoperative day 4. Before its

**Table 3–2** Nursing Care Plan: Multiple Trauma

| Patient Problem | Patient Goals | Target Date | Nursing Actions |
|---|---|---|---|
| Shock related to decreased blood volume and change in systemic vasculature | The patient will have no indication of shock as evidenced by<br><br>• hemodynamic values within normal limits<br>• mean arterial pressure, 70–90 mm Hg<br>• pulmonary artery pressure, 10–25/0–12 mm Hg<br>• pulmonary capillary wedge pressure, 0–12 mm Hg<br>• cardiac output, 4–8 liters/min<br>• cardiac index, 2.5–4 liters/min/m²<br>• systemic vascular resistance, 950–1,300 dyne-sec/cm⁻⁵<br>• pulmonary vascular resistance, 155–255 dyne-sec/cm⁻⁵<br>• heart rate, < 100/min and in sinus rhythm<br>• blood gas values within normal limits<br>• $PaO_2$, 80–100<br>• $PaCO_2$, 35–45<br>• pH, 7.35–7.45<br>• $O_2$%sat, 95–100%<br>• urine output > 30 ml/hour | Day of surgery | The nurse will<br><br>• continually monitor and notify physician of abnormalities in<br>• heart rate<br>• pulmonary artery pressure<br>• pulmonary capillary wedge pressure<br>• mean arterial pressure<br>• measure every 8 hours and as ordered<br>• cardiac output<br>• cardiac index<br>• systemic vascular resistance<br>• pulmonary vascular resistance and notify physician of abnormalities<br>• monitor and record blood gas values as ordered; notify physician of abnormalities<br>• measure and record all fluid loss: urine output, estimated blood loss, nasogastric drainage, stool<br>• notify physician of alterations in clinical assessment: presence of cyanosis, cool skin, diaphoresis, |

| | | | |
|---|---|---|---|
| | | | pulmonary rales, neck vein distention, or altered neurologic status |
| | | | • notify physician of urine output < 30 ml/hour |
| | | | • have replacement blood and fluids readily available if needed |
| | | | • maintain patent airway |
| | | | • monitor, record, and notify physician of abnormalities in pertinent laboratory studies, including hematocrit, hemoglobin, and chemistry profile |

• clinical examination
  • skin warm and dry
  • neurologically intact
  • absence of cyanosis, pulmonary congestion, or neck vein distention

| Potential infection related to | The patient will be free of infection as evidenced by | Day of surgery | In an effort to prevent infection, the nurse will |
|---|---|---|---|
| • invasive lines and monitoring devices<br>  • arterial line<br>  • pulmonary artery catheter<br>  • peripheral IVs<br>  • Foley catheter<br>• breaks in skin barrier because of traumatic injury and surgical repair<br>• overall hypermetabolic state | • no signs of wound infection, such as<br>  • edema<br>  • warmth<br>  • pain<br>  • redness<br>  • drainage<br>• no signs of sepsis, such as<br>  • fever<br>  • chills<br>  • diaphoresis<br>  • change in level of consciousness<br>• no signs of pulmonary infection, such as | | • monitor, record, and notify physician of any alteration in<br>  • body temperature<br>  • heart rate<br>  • respiration rate<br>  • blood pressure and mean arterial pressure<br>  • level of consciousness<br>• notify physician of any sign of infection, either wound, sepsis, pulmonary, or urinary<br>• monitor IV insertion sites<br>• labeling IV tubing and site with date and time of insertion |

**Table 3–2** continued

| Patient Problem | Patient Goals | Target Date | Nursing Actions |
|---|---|---|---|
| | • fever<br>• change in sputum<br>• altered blood gas values<br>• pulmonary congestion<br>• no signs of urinary tract infection, such as<br> • dysuria<br> • cloudy urine<br> • flank pain<br> • hematuria | | • rotating peripheral IV sites at least every 3 days<br>• observing IV sites for signs of infection and notifying physician if any such signs appear<br>• maintain aseptic technique when suctioning patient's oral airway; changing IV dressings, site, or tubing; and manipulating any invasive line or tubing<br>• maintain vigorous pulmonary toilette for patient:<br> • turn, cough, and deep breathing exercises every 2 hours<br> • vibropercussion and incentive spirometry as ordered |
| Impaired nutritional status related to increased nutritional demands and decreased nutritional intake | The patient will maintain adequate nutritional status as evidenced by<br>• blood urea nitrogen (BUN), 10–20 mg/dl<br>• serum glucose level, 70–110 mg/dl<br>• no physical signs of fatty acid deficiency, such as<br> • dry, scaly skin | Day of surgery | In an effort to maintain an adequate nutritional status, the nurse will<br>• monitor and report signs of increased BUN:<br> • vomiting<br> • lethargy<br> • headache<br> • abnormal serum BUN |

- weight loss > 10% of normal body weight
- increased heart rate
- no signs of electrolyte imbalance, such as
  - tremors
  - muscle cramping
  - irritability
- cardiac dysrhythmias related to electrolyte levels

- monitor and report signs of abnormal glucose levels, such as
  - confusion, lethargy, disorientation
  - abnormal serum glucose
- monitor and report any sign of fatty acid deficiency
- monitor and report signs of electrolyte imbalance
- weigh patient daily and record weight
- maintain accurate records of patient's intake and output
- observe patient for cardiac dysrhythmias
- as soon as patient is able to tolerate intake by mouth, have patient participate in planning diet to encourage intake

removal, however, a final hemodynamic profile was done (see Table 3–1).

Appropriate management of the varying physiologic alterations in multiple trauma patients requires detailed hemodynamic assessment and monitoring. Over the last few years, many advances have been made in hemodynamic monitoring capabilities. Direct and indirect parameters are now commonly measured, providing needed information for patient treatment. In the case of Mr. H, the use of sophisticated monitoring equipment, expertly trained clinical practitioners, and rapid intervention prevented him from becoming another highway statistic.

Mr. H was transferred from the ICU on postoperative day 5. His blood pressure and mean arterial pressure were stable. Hematocrit on the morning of transfer was 43.2 percent. Bowel sounds were hypoactive, and it was planned that nasogastric suction, with the patient receiving nothing by mouth, would continue another 12 to 24 hours.

## NURSING DIAGNOSIS AND CARE PLAN

The nursing staff developed a plan of care for Mr. H when he was admitted to the ICU (Table 3–2). The nursing diagnoses identified for Mr. H can be applied to most patients who have sustained multiple trauma, as well as to many surgical patients.

---

NOTES

1. Charles F. Frey, "Accidents and Trauma Care—1983," *Surgery Annual* 16 (1984): 69–89.

2. N. Thomas Ryan, "Metabolic Adaptations for Energy Production during Trauma and Sepsis," *Surgical Clinics of North America:* 56 (October 1976): 1073–1090.

3. Malcolm O. Perry, "Metabolic Response to Trauma," in *Care of the Trauma Patient,* ed. G.T. Shires (New York: McGraw-Hill, 1979), 62–74.

4. Donald S. Gann and Joseph F. Amaral, "The Pathophysiology of Trauma and Shock," in *The Management of Trauma,* ed. George D. Zuidema, Robert B. Rutherford, and William T. Ballinger (Philadelphia: W.B. Saunders, 1979), 37–103.

5. Christian J. Lambertsen, "Transport of Oxygen, Carbon Dioxide, and Inert Gases by the Blood," in *Medical Physiology,* 14th ed., ed. Vernon B. Montcastle (St. Louis: C.V. Mosby, 1980), 1721–1748.

6. Gann and Amaral, "Pathophysiology of Trauma and Shock," 1979.

7. Donald D. Trunkey, George F. Sheldon, and John A. Collins, "The Treatment of Shock," in *The Management of Trauma,* ed. George D. Zuidema, Robert B. Rutherford, and William T. Ballinger (Philadelphia: W.B. Saunders, 1979), 80–101.

8. William R. Milnor, "The Cardiovascular Control System," in *Medical Physiology,* 14th ed., ed. Vernon B. Montcastle (St. Louis: C.V. Mosby, 1980), 1061–1084.

9. John M. Haas, "Understanding Hemodynamic Monitoring: Concepts of Preload and Afterload," *Critical Care Quarterly 2* (September 1979): 1–8.

10. Trunkey, Sheldon, and Collins, "Treatment of Shock," 1979.

11. Milnor, "Cardiovascular Control System," 1980.

12. Haas, "Concepts of Preload and Afterload," 1979.

13. Ryan, "Energy Production during Trauma and Sepsis," 1976.

14. Perry, "Metabolic Response to Trauma," 1979.

15. Trunkey, Sheldon, and Collins, "Treatment of Shock," 1979.

16. Douglas W. Wilmore and Louis H. Aulick, "Systemic Response to Injury and the Healing Wound," *Journal of Parenteral and Enteral Nutrition* 4 (1980): 147–150.

17. Lambertsen, "Transport of Oxygen," 1980.

18. William R. Milnor, "Pulmonary Circulation," in *Medical Physiology,* 14th ed., ed. Vernon B. Montcastle (St. Louis: C.V. Mosby, 1980), 1108–1117.

19. Mary M. Hall, "Pros and Cons of Medical Anti-Shock Trousers," *Journal of Emergency Nursing* 11 (January/February 1985): 22–26.

20. Ronald D. Stewart, "Pre Hospital Care of Trauma," *Trauma Quarterly* 1 (May 1985): 1–13.

21. Haas, "Concepts of Preload and Afterload," 1979.

22. Mary W. Falconer et al., *The Drug, The Nurse, The Patient* (Philadelphia: W.B. Saunders, 1978).

23. William M. Stahl, "Crystalloid Versus Colloid Resuscitation," *Trauma Quarterly* (May 1985): 15–22.

24. Marilyn T. Haupt and Eric C. Rachow, "Colloid Osmotic Pressure and Fluid Resuscitation with Hetastarch, Albumin, and Saline Solutions," *Critical Care Medicine* 10 (March 1982): 159–162.

# Chapter 4

# Cardiac Transplantation

*Reba Felks-McVay, R.N., M.S.N.*

Patients considered for cardiac transplantation usually have end-stage heart disease, in which the contractility of the ventricles is poor. The primary diagnoses of the 62 cardiac transplant recipients at the University of Alabama in Birmingham from November, 1981, to July, 1985, were cardiomyopathy (42), ischemic heart disease (17), and congenital heart disease (3). The cause of the disease in a given patient may not be known, and the course of illness varies from one patient to another. Hospitalization may be necessary before transplantation to treat low cardiac output, congestive heart failure, and arrhythmias.

Donna M was a 33-year-old white woman who had been in relatively good health until 3 months earlier. She was married and had three children, aged 14, 9, and 5. Mrs. M went to see her physician when she became ill with a cough, sinus congestion, sore throat, and a temperature of 102°F for 2 days. Following the examination, the physician diagnosed her condition as an upper respiratory tract infection. Mrs. M was given appropriate treatment. Two weeks later, Mrs. M returned to see her physician because the cough was persistent and she was having difficulty breathing. Mrs. M, who had weighed 90 kg on her first visit, had lost 3 kg and was sleeping poorly. She stated that she was awakened often by coughing. The results of laboratory tests and urinalysis were all within normal limits, but her chest roentgenogram showed bilateral congestion and an increase in the size of her heart. Mrs. M was admitted to the hospital; her vital signs at this point are shown in Table 4–1. After diagnostic studies, her condition was diagnosed as congestive cardiomyopathy secondary to a viral infection.

Despite medication to decrease the severity of her congestive heart failure, Mrs. M's condition deteriorated over the next 8 weeks. She was transferred to a medical center for cardiac transplant evaluation. Mrs. M

**Table 4–1**  Donna M: Vital Signs

| Parameter | Admission Values | Pretransplant Values |
|---|---|---|
| Blood pressure | 110/70 mm Hg | 80/40–100/50 mm Hg |
| Heart rate | 100, normal sinus rhythm | 114, frequent premature ventricular contractions |
| Respiration rate | 20, labored | 24, work of breathing |
| Temperature | 98.8°F | 97.4°F |
| Pedal pulses | 3/3, warm, pink | 0/0, cool, pale |
| Weight | 87 kg | 72 kg |

was found to be an acceptable candidate for transplantation, and the search for a donor heart was begun.

Mrs. M's condition stabilized with the use of furosemide (Lasix), 100 mg twice each day; metolazone (Zaroxolyn), 5 mg daily; digoxin, 0.25 mg daily; and a potassium supplement. As her cardiac reserves diminished, Mrs. M required the addition of a dopamine drip at 5 μg/kg/min and a dobutamine drop at 2.5 μg/kg/min to maintain her systolic blood pressure higher than 100 mm Hg.

On the day of her transplant, Mrs. M's condition was stable, but the progression of her disease was evident. Her vital signs at this time are also shown in Table 4–1.

## HEMODYNAMIC MONITORING FOR CARDIAC TRANSPLANT RECIPIENTS

Like any patient who undergoes open heart surgery, the cardiac transplant recipient returns to the intensive care unit with an endotracheal tube for mechanical ventilation, epicardial pacing wires, lines for intracardiac pressure monitoring, two or more mediastinal chest tubes for drainage, an arterial line for blood pressure monitoring, a urinary catheter, and several intravenous (IV) lines. As soon as the patient arrives in the intensive care unit, electrodes are placed on the chest for monitoring heart rate and rhythm, and a probe is inserted rectally for monitoring body temperature.

The intracardiac pressures monitored are usually the right atrial pressure, pulmonary artery pressure, pulmonary capillary wedge pressure, and left atrial pressure. The systolic, diastolic, and mean arterial pressures are also monitored. The cardiac output and cardiac index are obtained by use of these monitoring lines.

The transplant patient is placed in a private room that has been thoroughly cleaned for strict reverse isolation. The machinery and equipment used are thoroughly cleaned or sterilized. Special care is taken to prevent contamination of all invasive lines, tubes, and devices. Anyone who enters the patient care area must wear cap, mask, gown, gloves, and booties. Cultures of urine and sputum are obtained weekly. These procedures are intended to protect the immunosuppressed patient from possible infection.

Both invasive and noninvasive parameters, such as cardiac function, perfusion, and circulating volume, are assessed in the cardiac transplant patient much as they are assessed in the cardiovascular surgical patient. The postoperative complications that may follow cardiovascular surgery, such as hemorrhage and tamponade, may also be seen after cardiac transplantation. Hemodynamic monitoring after cardiac transplantation is useful in the assessment of ischemic damage that may have occurred with procurement, responses to preexisting elevations in pulmonary vascular resistance, and the effects of residual organ system dysfunction, primarily renal and hepatic dysfunction.

**Assessment of Cardiac Function**

The transplanted heart must overcome insult caused by ischemia and cooling during the procurement process, reperfusion, and cardiopulmonary bypass. Studies have shown that myocardial depression follows transplantation, but that function is recovered within 3 days to near normal levels.[1,2] Cardiac output remains at low normal levels, however, and increased demands are met by the Frank-Starling mechanism (i.e., an increase in left ventricular end-diastolic volume).[3] Circulating catecholamines play an important role in the inotropic and chronotropic response of the denervated, transplanted heart.[4] The heart rate may be low immediately after surgery, but it rapidly increases and remains at above normal resting levels.[5] Determinations of cardiac output, cardiac index, right atrial pressure, pulmonary capillary wedge pressure (or left atrial pressure), blood pressure, heart rate, and rhythm are useful in assessing the function and recovery of the transplanted heart. The quality of pedal pulses, skin temperature and color, and urinary output are useful noninvasive methods of assessing tissue perfusion.

**Assessment of Pulmonary Vascular Response**

Preexisting elevations in the pulmonary vascular resistance affect the function of the right ventricle of the transplanted heart postoperatively.[6] The pulmonary vascular resistance and pulmonary pressures are evaluated during the preoperative period by right ventricle catheterization or monitoring of right ventricle pressures by Swan-Ganz catheter. If the pulmonary vascular resistance is low, no elevation in the pressure of the right ventricle is needed to push blood forward. If pulmonary disease has increased vascular resistance, however, the right side of the heart must compensate. Right ventricle failure occurs if the compensatory mechanisms cannot be activated within a few seconds or minutes.

It is useful to compare right atrial pressure with left atrial pressure in assessing and managing the right ventricular response to pulmonary pressure elevation.

## Assessment of Residual Organ System Dysfunction

The preoperative cardiac disease may have compromised other organ systems, not only causing dysfunction in these vital organ systems, but also damaging them. The renal, hepatic, and pulmonary systems must be observed closely in cardiac transplant recipients to assess the possibility of residual dysfunction and irreversible damage. Hemodynamic monitoring is of limited use in this assessment. Determinations of urinary output, BUN, and creatinine level; liver function studies; arterial blood gas analysis; and chest roentgenograms are more useful in assessing the function of these organ systems. If the transplant patient should develop a dysfunction that requires treatment, such as dialysis or hemofiltration, hemodynamic monitoring is used to assess the effect of treatment on the cardiovascular system. Because many of the medications used for immunosuppression and in the treatment of hypertension and infection are nephrotoxic or hepatotoxic, the function of the kidneys and liver must be assessed on a routine basis.

## Assessment during Rejection and Infection

Hemodynamic monitoring of cardiac transplant patients is not routinely necessary during the treatment of rejection or infection. If the transplant recipient becomes hemodynamically compromised, invasive monitoring is used in assessing the ability of the cardiovascular system to function and respond to treatment. Such an assessment is most likely to be done by means of a Swan-Ganz catheter and an arterial line. Cardiac transplant patients who require hemodynamic monitoring are transferred to the intensive care unit for close observation.

On admission to the intensive care unit, Mrs. M's endotracheal tube was connected to an intermittent mandatory ventilation ventilator with the settings at intermittent mandatory ventilation 10, fraction of inspired oxygen ($FiO_2$) 60 percent, tidal volume 700, and positive end expiratory pressure (PEEP) +4 cm. Bilateral breath sounds could be auscultated. Electrocardiogram (ECG) electrodes were placed on her chest in a standard lead II position, and normal sinus rhythm with a rate of 60 beats/min appeared on the scope. The intracardiac monitoring lines and arterial line were connected to transducers for monitoring. The two mediastinal chest tubes were connected to a bedside bottle with a water seal and wall suction for drainage. Her Foley catheter was attached to a bedside drainage bag for hourly measurement, and a rectal temperature probe was inserted. Mrs. M's pedal pulses were 3/3; her skin was cold and its color pale. A hypothermia blanket was placed on the bed to provide the warmth that Mrs. M needed after surgery. Mrs. M's hemodynamic parameters are listed in Table 4–2. Mrs. M was placed in strict reverse isolation in the intensive care unit. Special care was taken to prevent contamination of all invasive lines, devices, and tubes.

Mrs. M appeared to be in stable condition following cardiac transplantation. There were no signs of ischemic damage or right ventricular failure. The hemodynamic pressures were within acceptable limits, and cardiac function appeared to be adequate. Mrs. M's renal function was more than satisfactory, as her urinary output remained higher than 100 ml/hour. Laboratory studies were ordered to evaluate her liver and renal function.

## GOALS AND MANAGEMENT

The cardiac transplant recipient is usually monitored hemodynamically until the third or fourth postoperative day. With stabilization of cardiac and pulmonary function, intracardiac pressures approach those found in stable well-functioning hearts. Cardiac output is in the low normal range, and the heart rate is higher than normal resting levels. The increases in blood pressure that follow transplantation

**Table 4–2** Hemodynamic Parameters of Mrs. M after Cardiac Transplantation

| | *Time* | | | | | |
|---|---|---|---|---|---|---|
| *Parameters* | *3:00* | *3:30* | *4:00* | *4:30* | *5:00* | *6:00* |
| Right atrial pressure (mm Hg) | 5 | 6 | 7 | 5 | 5 | 6 |
| Pulmonary artery-systolic | 50 | 45 | 44 | 48 | 50 | 48 |
| Pulmonary artery-diastolic | 20 | 22 | 19 | 18 | 21 | 20 |
| Left atrial pressure | 10 | 12 | 12 | 11 | 10 | 12 |
| Systolic blood pressure (mm Hg) | 120 | 131 | 154 | 126 | 118 | 125 |
| Diastolic blood pressure | 54 | 66 | 77 | 60 | 50 | 59 |
| Mean arterial pressure | 70 | 84 | 100 | 77 | 68 | 77 |
| Heart rate (beats/min) | 60 | 85 | 85 | 85 | 85 | 85 |
| Respiration rate | 10 | 10 | 10 | 10 | 10 | 12 |
| Temperature (°C) | 33.8 | 34.5 | 36 | 37 | 37.4 | 37.4 |
| Urine (ml/hour) | 150 | 200 | 200 | 500 | 300 | 300 |
| Chest drainage (ml/hour) | 75 | 70 | 50 | 50 | 50 | 50 |
| Cardiac output | | 6.08 | | | | 5.60 |
| Cardiac index | | 2.83 | | | | 1.90 |
| Pedal pulses | 3/3 | 3/3 | 3/3 | 3/3 | 3/3 | 2/2 |

may be attributed to the use of cyclosporine. The manipulations of cardiovascular parameters to optimize cardiac function are very similar to those used after any cardiac surgery.

In the presence of a low preload, for example, leukocyte-poor blood, whole blood, packed red blood cells, or albumin may be infused to elevate the left atrial pressure or the pulmonary capillary wedge pressure to optimal levels. The treatment of elevated preload may include the use of diuretics, such as Lasix, mannitol, or Zaroxolyn. If the left atrial pressure or pulmonary capillary wedge pressure rises above 18 or 20 mm Hg, vasodilators, such as sodium nitroprusside (Nipride) or nitroglycerine, may be infused to keep pressures at a lower level.

The manipulation of afterload can be monitored by measurements of systolic blood pressure, mean arterial pressure, or systemic vascular resistance. The drugs of choice for the treatment of an elevated afterload are Nipride or nitroglycerine infusions. When a cardiac transplant patient has a low afterload, the most appropriate intervention is to diagnose and treat the underlying cause. Vasopressors are rarely, if ever, used in the postoperative care of the cardiac transplant recipient.

Because the denervated heart is more sensitive to circulating catecholamines and responds appropriately to demands for an increase in cardiac output, positive inotropic agents can be used to support and improve contractile force and cardiac output in the immediate postoperative period. The catecholamines most commonly used are isoproterenol (Isuprel), dopamine, and dobutamine. The cardiac output and cardiac index, as well as hemodynamic pressures, pedal pulses, skin temperature and color, neurologic function, and urinary output, are monitored every 4 hours.

The heart rate may be low initially, but it increases to 80 to 110 beats/min within 3 to 4 days after transplantation. Junctional rhythms, premature ventricular contractions, atrioventricular blocks, and atrial arrhythmias may be observed in the immediate postoperative period when ischemia, electrolyte imbalances, and tissue edema are resolving. The sinus node of the recipient heart may have been left intact in the remaining atria; although it does not stimulate the donor heart, its electrical activity is recorded on the ECG as an extra P wave. Epicardial pacing wires attached to the donor right atrium and right ventricle are used for temporary pacing to override arrhythmias and to increase heart rate.

During the first 20 minutes in intensive care, Mrs. M developed a junctional rhythm with a heart rate of 55 beats/min. A temporary pacemaker was attached to her epicardial pacing wires and atrial asynchronous pacing at a rate of 85 beats/min was initiated. Cardiac output was measured when her temperature reached 34°C. Mrs. M was found to have a cardiac output of 6.08 liters/min and a cardiac index of 2.83 liters/min/m$^2$ (see Table 4–2).

Although her left atrial pressure was within normal limits, leukocyte-poor blood was administered to increase preload and to treat a hemoglobin of 8.5 g/dl. The left atrial pressure was at a range of 12 to 14 mm Hg. With the improvement of her cardiac function and increased blood flow, Mrs. M's pulmonary artery pressure decreased to a range of 40 to 48/17 to 23 mm Hg. Her pedal pulses remained at 3/3 with her skin cool and color pale.

As Mrs. M began to awaken, her blood pressure increased to a systolic pressure of 150 to 160 mm Hg. An infusion of Nipride was titrated to maintain her systolic blood pressure within the range of 120 to 130 mm Hg. Mrs. M appeared to be anxious, and she was given morphine intravenously to help her relax and to relieve possible pain. When she relaxed, a cardiac output with index was obtained. The cardiac output was 5.60 liters/min, and the cardiac index was 1.90 liters/min/m². Intracardiac pressures were within acceptable levels, and her blood pressure was stable. Her pedal pulses were found to be 2/2; her skin was cool and pale. An infusion of dopamine was started at 2.5 μg/kg/min to increase cardiac output. Within 10 minutes, Mrs. M had pedal pulses of 3/3, and her skin was cool and pink. Urinary output remained more than 100 ml/hour.

The management of the cardiac transplant patient is very similar to that of the cardiac surgical patient. The invasive monitoring lines and devices are removed by the second or third postoperative day in order to decrease the risk of contamination and infection. The patient is rapidly returned to routine activities of daily living, and rehabilitation is planned according to the patient's needs. The patient receives information about medications, diet, exercise, and home care. In order to detect any signs of rejection, routine right ventricular endomyocardial biopsies are performed every 5 to 7 days while the patient is in the hospital. The patient is returned home able to resume normal activities. Many return to work or school within months of transplantation.

Mrs. M's condition stabilized, and she was extubated within 6 hours of surgery. Her invasive monitoring lines were removed on the second postoperative day, and ambulation was begun in the isolation room. On the third day following transplantation, Mrs. M was transferred to a private room on the surgical ward to begin learning how to care for herself at home and rebuilding muscle strength. She returned home to her family just 8 weeks after transplantation with no complications.

**Table 4–3** Nursing Care Plan: Cardiac Transplantation

| Patient Problem | Patient Goals | Target Date | Nursing Actions |
|---|---|---|---|
| Potential hemodynamic alterations secondary to | The patient will maintain adequate hemodynamics as evidenced by | Day of surgery | The nurse will |
| • ischemia during procurement | • hemodynamic parameters within normal limits | | • continuously monitor |
| • denervation | • heart rate > 85 with normal sinus rhythm | | • intracardiac pressures |
| • myocardial depression | | | • arterial blood pressure |
| • reperfusion | • systolic blood pressure, 100–140 mm Hg | | • heart rate |
| • preexisting elevated pulmonary vascular resistance | • mean arterial pressure, 60–95 mm Hg | | • rhythm |
| • cardiopulmonary bypass | • right atrial pressure, 3–7 mm Hg | | • monitor and record every 30 minutes: pedal pulses, skin temperature and color, pupillary reaction or neurologic status |
| | • left atrial pressure, 10–14 mm Hg | | • monitor and record hourly: urinary output and chest tube drainage |
| | • pulmonary artery pressure-systolic, 20–30 mm Hg | | • measure cardiac output and index every 4 hours and as needed; report to physician cardiac index less than $2.0$ liters/min/m$^2$ |
| | • cardiac index > $2.04$ liters/min/m$^2$ | | |
| | • right atrial pressure < left atrial pressure | | • monitor preload, afterload, heart rate, and contractility; intervene as ordered |
| | • color and perfusion adequate by assessment of | | • report to physician any changes in hemodynamic parameters |
| | • pedal pulses > +2 | | • insulate pacing wires and secure temporary pacemaker to bed for possible use |
| | • skin pink and warm | | |
| | • urine output > 30 ml/hour | | |
| | • neurologic status intact | | |

Potential rejection of transplanted heart

The patient will experience no rejection as evidenced by

- right ventricular endomyocardial biopsy free of evidence of rejection
- hemodynamics within normal limits on right ventricular catheterization, such as
  - right atrial pressure, 3–7 mm Hg
  - pulmonary artery pressure, 20–30/10–12 mm Hg
  - pulmonary capillary wedge pressure, 5–12 mm Hg
  - cardiac index, > 2.0 liters/min/m$^2$
  - heart rate > 85 beats/min without ectopy
  - systolic blood pressure, 100–130 mm Hg
- color and perfusion adequate as assessed by
  - pedal pulses > +2
  - skin pink and warm
  - urinary output > 30 ml/hour
  - neurologic status intact
- no signs or symptoms of rejection, such as
  - lethargy
  - mood swings
  - edema or weight gain

The nurse will

- observe for signs and symptoms of rejection, such as
  - lethargy
  - mood swings
  - edema or weight gain
  - heart sounds S3, S4
  - atrial or ventricular arrhythmias
  - decreased exercise tolerance
  - decreased pedal pulses
  - work of breathing, shortness of breath, jugular vein distention, normalization of blood pressure
  - decreased ECG voltage
  - fever
  - joint pain
- obtain vital signs (i.e., blood pressure, heart rate, respiration rate and pedal pulses) every 4 hours
- observe and document ECG for arrhythmias
- obtain daily weight
- record strict intake and output
- obtain daily ECG for 3 days, then every Monday
- prepare patient for biopsy; explain and obtain permit for procedure; give nothing by mouth before biopsy

**Table 4-3** continued

| Patient Problem | Patient Goals | Target Date | Nursing Actions |
|---|---|---|---|
| | • S3, S4, jugular vein distention<br>• atrial or ventricular arrhythmias<br>• decreased exercise tolerance<br>• decreased pedal pulses<br>• shortness of breath<br>• normalization of blood pressure<br>• decreased ECG voltage (azathioprine [Imuran])<br>• fever<br>• joint pain | | • following biopsy, observe for<br>    • pneumothorax<br>    • hemothorax<br>    • bleeding at biopsy site<br>    • edema or hematoma at biopsy site<br>• administer medications to treat rejection as ordered; observe for reactions |
| Potential infection secondary to immunosuppression | The patient will experience no infection as evidenced by<br><br>• temperature < 100°F<br>• white blood count, 5,000–10,000<br>• platelet count, 150,000–300,000<br>• chest roentgenogram clear<br>• wounds healing without redness, edema, or drainage<br>• sputum clear<br>• results of sputum and urine cultures negative<br>• no oral lesions<br>• no nausea/vomiting or diarrhea<br>• no headache<br>• no sinus congestion | | The nurse will<br><br>• observe proper isolation technique (i.e., use of gown, mask, gloves, booties, hat)<br>• provide sterile care of wounds, tubes, devices, in-dwelling lines<br>• not allow those with contagious disease to enter transplant room<br>• provide Foley catheter care every 8 hours or as needed<br>• ensure sterile care of endotracheal tube<br>• monitor body temperature continuously for 72 hours, then every 4 hours or as needed<br>• obtain daily complete blood count with differential and platelet count |

- obtain daily chest roentgenogram for 2 weeks
- provide wound care every 8 hours or as needed; observe for drainage, redness, tenderness
- obtain weekly sputum and urine cultures
- examine sputum when obtainable; note color, consistency, amount
- observe for symptoms, such as
  - nausea
  - vomiting
  - diarrhea
  - headache
  - stiff neck
  - painful breathing
  - cough
  - sore throat
  - sniffles
  - sinus congestion
- alert physician to abnormal temperature, laboratory results, or symptoms of possible infection

## NURSING DIAGNOSIS AND CARE PLAN

Although the immediate postoperative care plan written for Mrs. M (Table 4–3) pertains to the cardiac transplant recipient, it can also be used for the recipient of a heart and lung transplant. The nursing diagnosis regarding the potential for infection in the immunosuppressed patient, observations, and nursing actions can be used in caring for any immunosuppressed patient, such as patients who are receiving chemotherapy or who have undergone any organ transplantation.

**NOTES**

1. J.S. Schroeder, "Hemodynamic Performance of the Human Transplanted Heart," *Transplantation Proceedings* 11 (March 1979):304–308.
2. Michael L. Hess et al., "Mechanical and Subcellular Function of the Canine Heterotopic Transplanted Myocardium during Active Transplant Injury," *Transplantation* 32 (September 1981):194–202.
3. Michael DeBakey et al., "Human Cardiac Transplantation: Clinical Experience," *Journal of Thoracic and Cardiovascular Surgery* 58 (September 1969):303–317.
4. Richard A. Carleton et al., "Hemodynamic Performance of a Transplanted Human Heart," *Circulation* 40 (October 1969):447–452.
5. Edward B. Stinson et al., "Hemodynamic Observations One and Two Years after Cardiac Transplantation in Man," *Circulation* 45 (June 1972):1183–1194.
6. Grady L. Hallman et al., "Function of the Transplanted Human Heart," *Journal of Thoracic and Cardiovascular Surgery* 58 (September 1969):318–325.

**REFERENCES**

Beck, W., Barnard, C.N., and Schrire, V. "Heart Rate after Cardiac Transplantation." *Circulation* 40 (1969):437–445.

Bexton, Rodney S., et al. "Electrophysiological Abnormalities in the Transplanted Human Heart." *British Heart Journal* 50(1983):555–563.

McLaughlin, Peter R., et al. "The Effect of Exercise and Atrial Pacing on LV Volume and Contractility in Patients with Innervated and Denervated Hearts." *Circulation* 58(1978):476–483.

# Chapter 5

# Sepsis

*Nancy Reeder, R.N., M.S.N., C.C.R.N.*

The clinical syndrome of sepsis has become a widely recognized cause of morbidity and mortality in critically ill patients. Sepsis is generally a hospital-acquired syndrome that develops secondary to treatment or events during hospitalization. Certain patient groups, such as the very young or the very old, are compromised hosts. Other host-related factors are malnutrition, general debilitation, and chronic health problems (e.g., hepatic dysfunction, cardiac disease, renal disease, diabetes, and alcoholism). Invasive medical procedures, chemical or endogenous immunosuppression, widespread use of antibiotics, and traumatic injuries also predispose the critically ill patient to sepsis.[1] Whatever the etiology or risk factors, sepsis is one of the most dreaded complications of critical illness.

There are different clinical states within the syndrome of sepsis. Sepsis itself is defined as a systemic response to invading organisms. Bacteremia is the presence of bacteria in the bloodstream. These bacteria may or may not be alive and multiplying; there may or may not be pathophysiologic changes.[2] Frequently, removal of the cause (e.g., an invasive device) resolves the symptoms. Bacteremia does not always lead to septicemia, which is a severe infection caused by the presence of rapidly multiplying bacteria in the bloodstream.

The culmination of these states is septic shock. In this final state, cellular function is impaired and hemodynamics altered. Despite increased understanding of the pathophysiology, the mortality rate associated with septic shock is higher than is that associated with either cancer or traumatic injury secondary to auto accidents.[3] A 40 to 90 percent mortality rate is associated with septic shock.[4,5]

## PHYSIOLOGIC IMPLICATIONS OF SEPSIS

Septic shock causes catastrophic changes in the metabolic, cardiovascular, pulmonary, renal, hepatic, and gastrointestinal systems. The development of a diabeteslike state is one of the most profound changes. Hyperglycemia develops secondary to a decrease in insulin production and an increase in cellular resistance to circulating insulin. The cells become unable to use first glucose, then fat, and finally protein as an energy source.[6] Alterations in glucose and fat metabolism impair the ability of the liver to use these substances, and protein catabolism increases. The end result is that, because of the liver's inability to use the amino acids, the blood levels of nitrogenous wastes and amino acids increase.

Various hormonal secretions are increased during sepsis. Adrenocorticotropic hormone (ACTH) secretion stimulates cortisol secretion from the adrenal cortex. Secretion of cortisol stimulates glyconeogenesis to provide higher levels of glucose for metabolic needs. The posterior pituitary gland increases its secretion of the antidiuretic hormone (ADH) during stress, resulting in water retention and, potentially, oliguria. Secretion of the hormone aldosterone from the adrenal cortex leads to increased sodium reabsorption and, thus, increased fluid retention. Both of these latter hormones act to maintain the intravascular volume.

The sympathetic nervous system responds to sepsis by increasing the secretion of catecholamines, particularly epinephrine.[7] These catecholamines increase the heart rate, blood pressure, and cardiac contractility. Other effects on the cardiovascular system are primarily β-adrenergic. Tachycardia, tachydysrhythmias, and elevated cardiac output in the face of normal blood volume are preliminary signs of septic shock.[8,9]

Significant changes also occur within the pulmonary system. Pulmonary blood flow decreases, and pulmonary vascular resistance rises to more than 250 dynes-sec/cm$^{-5}$. The release of endotoxins by the bacteria alters cellular membranes, increasing capillary permeability. As a result, fluid and protein leak from the pulmonary capillaries, and interstitial pulmonary edema occurs. Marked platelet aggregation in the pulmonary capillaries causes sludging and obstruction, leading to atelectasis. The leakage of protein into the alveoli inactivates surfactant, exacerbating atelectasis. Adult respiratory distress syndrome (ARDS) is a common sequela to these pulmonary derangements.

The renal system responds to decreased blood flow by activating the renin-angiotensin system. The ultimate result is the production of norepinephrine, which induces vasoconstriction to help maintain an adequate core arterial pressure. Aldosterone, which effects the conservation of sodium and, hence, water, is also secreted. Urine output drops. Unfortunately, prolonged vasoconstriction of the renal arteries may result in renal ischemia that may evolve into acute tubular necrosis.

The detoxifying functions of the hepatic system are severely impaired in the presence of sepsis. Disseminated intravascular coagulation and other consumptive coagulopathies develop when the liver can no longer synthesize appropriate clotting factors. Decreased perfusion of the liver also has a negative effect on the

production of glycogen and release of glucose, contributing to hyperglycemia.[10,11]

Because gastrointestinal vessels are constricted during shock, gastrointestinal
mucosa becomes ischemic, and fluid passes into the bowel lumen and ileus. This
fluid loss aggravates an already debilitating systemic fluid loss. Development of a
paralytic ileus may interfere not only with gastrointestinal function, but also with
ventilation, because it interferes with elevation of the diaphragm. Ischemia alters
cellular membranes by increasing their permeability to large molecules, such as
protein and bacteria. These patients are predisposed to stress ulcers and gastric
bleeding.[12]

The effects of septic shock on the cellular level are primarily due to the release
of endotoxins from the invading bacteria and the consequent release of chemicals
from cells damaged by the infectious process. Histamine and bradykinin are
released from the mast cells, causing vasodilation and contributing to increased
capillary permeability.[13] Because of the increased capillary permeability, protein
and fluid move from the capillaries to the interstitial space; this results in a relative
hypovolemia and buildup of lactic acid.

Another chemical released in late shock is myocardial depressant factor, or
myocardial toxic factor. This substance is a lysosomal hydrolase thought to be a
byproduct of the chemicals released from pancreatic cells after prolonged ischemia. Myocardial depressant factor produces severe negative inotropic responses
by depressing cardiac contractility and by interfering with calcium ion balance.[14]

The end result of the impaired tissue perfusion during septic shock is a decrease
in the intracellular oxygen levels. A decrease in ATP forces the cell to function
anaerobically so that it produces large amounts of lactic acid. As a result of the
ATP deficiency, sodium and water shift into the cell, while potassium and
magnesium shift out of the cell. With the influx of water, the cells swell, and
irreversible damage to the cell membrane and organelles occurs. Lysosomal
enzyme leakage into the cell causes cellular autodigestion.[15]

The question of whether cellular alterations are due to decreased oxygen
delivery or impaired oxygen use is controversial. Shires and associates concluded
from their studies that cells actually build up ATP and, thus, cellular alterations
result from impaired oxygen use.[16] Kaufman and associates, however, found that
increased oxygen delivery in early shock improves oxygen use at the cellular level;
they theorized that the problem may be selective vasoconstriction and hypovolemia. They suggested that intracellular blockade may be the problem in cellular
oxygen use during late shock.[17]

## ETIOLOGY

Septicemia is caused predominantly by gram-negative bacilli, less often by
gram-positive bacilli. Septicemia occurs in patients who have become compro-

mised hosts as a result of diseases or therapies that alter the body's normal immune defense mechanisms. There are four portals of entry (Table 5–1).

## HEMODYNAMIC MONITORING FOR PATIENTS WITH SEPSIS

Septic shock has two phases: hyperdynamic (warm) shock and hypodynamic (cold) shock. Hyperdynamic septic shock occurs while circulating blood volume is still adequate. These patients usually have dry skin and are warm, pink, and flushed. Peripheral arterial and venous vasodilation is a primary derangement; it results from the release of vasoactive substances, such as histamines and endorphins.[18] Vasodilation of the arterioles causes a drop in the systemic vascular resistance to less than 800 dynes-sec/cm$^{-5}$. The body's initial response to this decrease in the systemic vascular resistance is a drop in arterial blood pressure. In order to maintain an adequate blood pressure, the body then increases the cardiac output. Thus, the cardiac output remains normal or may even be elevated (4 to 8 liters/min). The venous system also dilates, producing venous pooling and, thus, decreasing venous return to the heart. In the warm phase of shock, decreased venous return does not appear to lower the cardiac output significantly. A reflex tachycardia partially compensates for this reduced venous return.

The relative hypovolemia that follows the fluid shifts to the interstitial space contributes to the development of hypodynamic septic shock. The cardiac output is decreased by alterations in heart rate, preload, afterload, and contractility. In response to a fall in the mean arterial pressure, the sympathetic nervous system causes peripheral vasoconstriction. The systemic vascular resistance rises to a level above 1,200 dynes-sec/cm$^{-5}$ in response to the vasoconstriction. Tachycardia causes a decrease in diastolic filling and coronary artery perfusion times. The presence of myocardial depressant factor, hypoxemia, acidosis, and endotoxins reduces cardiac contractility. The increase in systemic vascular resistance contributes to an increase in afterload. The patient becomes cold and clammy, and has mottled, cyanotic skin. Other classic signs of shock, such as weak and thready peripheral pulses, oliguria, and a reduced sensorium, become apparent.[19]

Mr. C was a 47-year-old white man who arrived in the intensive care unit after extensive surgery to repair damage from a gunshot wound to the abdomen. His medical history included hypertension, a duodenal ulcer, and probable alcohol abuse. The .38-caliber bullet had traversed his gallbladder, the left lobe of his liver, his pylorus, and his gastric antrum. Exploratory surgery included dissection of the liver lobe, cholecystectomy, insertion of a T tube for drainage of the common bile duct, and an axion pump to drain the gunshot wound entrance. His wound was considered clean at first, but it became contaminated

**Table 5–1** Portals of Entry for Bacteria

| | Common Mechanisms | Organisms | Comments |
|---|---|---|---|
| Urinary tract | Urinary catheterization<br>Cystoscopy | *Escherichia coli*<br>*Pseudomonas aeruginosa*<br>*Klebsiella-Enterobacter-Serratia*<br>(KES)<br>*Proteus* | Gram-negative bacteria enter here most often. |
| Respiratory tract | Open airways<br>Intubation<br>Tracheostomy<br>Ventilators<br>Suctioning<br>Bronchoscopy<br>Respiratory therapy | *E. coli*<br>*Pseudomonas*<br>KES<br>*Streptococcus pneumoniae*<br>*Staphylococcus* | Gram-negative organisms dominate inside the hospital.<br><br>Gram-positive organisms are the primary cause of pneumonias and bacteremias acquired outside the hospital. |
| Gastrointestinal tract | Surgery<br>Abscesses<br>Obstruction<br>Trauma causing organ rupture or perforation | *E. coli*<br>*Bacteroides*<br>KES<br>*Salmonella* | |
| Integumentary system | Burns<br>Abscesses<br>Parenteral therapy<br>Invasive lines and catheters | *Pseudomonas aeruginosa*<br>*Serratia*<br>*Acinetobacter*<br>*Staphylococcus* | As the body's first line of defense, violation of the skin has great potential for bacteremia. |

through spillage of ruptured organ contents into the peritoneal cavity. Initial resuscitative management included insertion of a Foley catheter (after negative intravenous pyelography), two large-bore peripheral lines, and a jugular central line; a Swan-Ganz catheter and arterial line were inserted during surgery. Hemodynamic parameters immediately after surgery revealed a low right atrial pressure and a low pulmonary capillary wedge pressure (Table 5–2).

For the first 4 days after surgery, treatment followed a typical pattern of volume replacement for a moderate blood loss because of surgery and abnormal hepatic clotting disorders. Mr. C was weaned from the ventilator, and he was eventually extubated. Hemodynamics stabilized as volume was replaced. The results of clotting studies were approaching normal. Because he experienced an isolated temperature spike to 102.2°F and because he was an exceptionally compromised host, cultures of his sputum, urine, wound, and blood were drawn. All were negative after 48 hours. Antibiotics were discontinued after 96 hours so that the invading organism could be identified and appropriate antibiotics ordered.

Postoperative day 5 marked a deterioration in Mr. C's condition. His temperature rose to 101.6°F, and he developed coarse rhonchi, yellow sputum, and tachypnea. Cultures of his sputum and drain site were again drawn. On postoperative day 6, Mr. C. became progressively more unresponsive, began hypoventilating, and was placed on the ventilator. During intubation, Mr. C vomited and aspirated the vomitus. The chest roentgenogram showed a progression of patchy infiltrates and an elevated right diaphragm. The diagnosis of aspiration pneumonia was made.

**Table 5–2** Mr. C: Hemodynamic Profiles

|  | Admission | Postoperative Day 4 |
|---|---|---|
| Heart rate | 125 | 98 |
| Mean arterial pressure | 75 mm Hg | 84 mm Hg |
| Right atrial pressure | 2 mm Hg | 6 mm Hg |
| Pulmonary artery pressure | 19/3 mm Hg | 23/10 mm Hg |
| Pulmonary capillary wedge pressure | 5 mm Hg | 11 mm Hg |
| Cardiac output | 4.3 liters/min | 5.6 liters/min |
| Systemic vascular resistance | 1,358 dynes-sec/cm$^{-5}$ | 1,114 dynes-sec/cm$^{-5}$ |
| Pulmonary vascular resistance | 62 dynes-sec/cm$^{-5}$ | 47 dynes-sec/cm$^{-5}$ |

By postoperative day 11, cultures were positive. *Pseudomonas aeruginosa* was growing in both his sputum and urine. Gram-positive rods, *Staphylococcus epidermidis,* were growing from his abdominal wound cultures; this was believed to be a true growth, not a skin contaminant. Tobramycin, clindamycin, cefotaxime sodium (claforan), and amphotericin B were administered. Blood cultures remained negative.

The following day, Mr. C's condition continued to deteriorate. Again his temperature spiked. This was accompanied by a marked decrease in urine output, a decrease in platelet count, and an increase in fibrin split products. The nephrologist who was consulted felt that the patient was becoming oliguric and that the probable cause was septicemia. A Swan-Ganz catheter was inserted, and the parameters obtained suggested development of warm shock. He was hyperdynamic with a cardiac output of 8.9 liters/min and a low systemic vascular resistance of 827 dynes-sec/cm$^{-5}$ (Table 5–3).

Medical management was directed toward the septicemia. Episodes of hypotension were alleviated with dopamine and volume replacement, when indicated. The oliguria and rising blood urea nitrogen (BUN) and creatinine levels were treated with hemodialysis. A bicarbonate drip was required to treat his lactic acidosis. An insulin drip ran continuously to control high serum glucose levels.

Within 24 hours, Mr. C's cardiac index dropped to 1.8 liters/min, and his systemic vascular resistance rose to 1,379 dynes-sec/cm$^{-5}$ (see Table 5–3). He was cool, pale, clammy, and tachycardic. His pulmonary picture reflected ARDS, and he became anuric. Disseminated intravascular coagulation was evident in his clotting studies and clinical

**Table 5–3** Mr. C: Hemodynamic Profiles in Shock

|  | *Hyperdynamic* | *Hypodynamic* |
|---|---|---|
| Heart rate | 136 | 144 |
| Mean arterial pressure | 100 mm Hg | 60 mm Hg |
| Right atrial pressure | 8 mm Hg | 10 mm Hg |
| Pulmonary artery pressure | 10/18 mm Hg | 49/20 mm Hg |
| Pulmonary capillary wedge pressure | 12 mm Hg | 21 mm Hg |
| Cardiac output | 8.9 liters/min | 2.9 liters/min |
| Systemic vascular resistance | 827 dynes-sec/cm$^{-5}$ | 1,379 dynes-sec/cm$^{-5}$ |
| Pulmonary vascular resistance | 119 dynes-sec/cm$^{-5}$ | 347 dynes-sec/cm$^{-5}$ |

assessment. Blood cultures demonstrated *S. epidermidis,* which was highly resistant to antibiotic therapy.

Treatment modalities were aimed at reducing preload and afterload with sodium nitroprusside (Nipride). Forward flow through the heart was augmented with the use of dopamine and, eventually, dobutamine. The goals were to reduce systemic vascular resistance and increase cardiac output. When volume status permitted, albumin was administered to draw fluid out of the extravascular space and into the intravascular space by increasing the plasma oncotic pressure. Daily hemodialysis was complicated by a consistently low mean arterial pressure.

Despite aggressive medical treatment of all of Mr. C's physiologic derangements, he died on postoperative day 20. Autopsy revealed the following: single gunshot wound involving primarily the liver and gallbladder, consumptive coagulopathy, renal failure, respiratory failure (ARDS), liver failure, malnutrition, and gastrointestinal hemorrhage. Death was attributed to septic shock.

Treatment modalities for a patient with septicemia are directed primarily at elimination of the cause of sepsis. Without aggressive treatment of the cause, treatment of the resulting symptoms is fruitless.

Hemodynamic monitoring of these patients gives valuable information about volume status and fluid shifts, vascular responses to circulating toxins, and the cumulative effects on cardiac output. It is necessary to achieve an adequate volume status in order to maintain an acceptable cardiac output. Manipulation may involve improving forward flow by reducing afterload with vasodilators. Reduction of afterload decreases the workload of the heart and oxygen demand. Concurrently, it may be necessary to use a dopaminergic agent to improve contractility and cardiac output. Small manipulations in drug and other treatment modalities allow the health care team to optimize hemodynamic therapy without excessive over- or undercompensation. Despite the fact that great strides have been made in the understanding and manipulation of measurable and derived hemodynamic parameters, the health care team can only maintain life while frantically attempting to treat the underlying problem: sepsis.

## NURSING DIAGNOSIS AND CARE PLAN

Excerpts from the nursing care plan for Mr. C are outlined in Table 5–4. Each nursing diagnosis addresses changes in volume status and its impact on hemodynamic parameters. Exhibit 5–1 is an example of a hemodynamic profile form for use in collecting data.

**Table 5–4** Nursing Care Plan: Sepsis

| Patient Problem | Patient Goals | Target Date | Nursing Actions |
|---|---|---|---|
| Admission: hypovolemia related to massive blood and fluid loss | Normovolemia as evidenced by<br><br>• normal sinus rhythm, > 60 < 100<br>• systolic blood pressure, > 90 < 150<br>• cardiac index, > 2.5 liters/min/m²<br>• pulmonary artery end-diastolic pressure, 8–15 mm Hg<br>• pulmonary capillary wedge pressure, 6–12 mm Hg<br>• urine output, > 20–30/ml/hour<br>• skin warm, dry, and pink<br>• peripheral pulses ≥ 2+<br>• normal sensorium | Within 24 hours of hypovolemia diagnosis | The nurse will<br><br>• monitor vital signs every 30 min and as required<br>• monitor pulmonary artery and pulmonary pressures every 12 hrs<br>• monitor capillary wedge pressures every 12 hours<br>• check peripheral pulses every 2 hours<br>• record hourly urine output measurements<br>• assess skin turgor and color, moistness of mucous membrane every 2 hours<br>• observe for signs of poor perfusion due to vasoconstriction:<br>  • slow nailbed capillary refill<br>  • pale or dusky nailbeds<br>  • cool or clammy extremities<br>• measure all drainage every 4 hours<br>• monitor hematocrit, potassium, sodium, BUN, and creatinine for signs of hemoconcentration |

**Table 5-4** Nursing Care Plan: Sepsis

| Patient Problem | Patient Goals | Target Date | Nursing Actions |
|---|---|---|---|
| Admission: hypovolemia related to massive blood and fluid loss | | | The nurse will<br>• if hypovolemia occurs<br>• administer as ordered volume expanders, such as blood or blood products, and vasopressors in conjunction with volume expanders<br>• elevate feet to increase venous return |
| Postoperative day 4: increased cardiac workload and oxygen consumption secondary to increased systemic vascular resistance | Systemic vascular resistance of 800–1200 dynes-sec/cm$^{-5}$<br>Absence of peripheral vasoconstriction as evidenced by<br>• full strong peripheral pulses bilaterally<br>• warm, pink, dry skin | Postoperative day 5 | The nurse will<br>• treat volume status with volume expanders as ordered if<br>• pulmonary capillary wedge pressure < 6<br>• pulmonary artery end-diastolic pressure < 8<br>• titrate vasodilator drips to keep systemic vascular resistance > 800 < 1,200 dynes-sec/cm$^{-5}$<br>• monitor hemodynamic profile every 4 hours when administering vasoactive drug therapy |

Postoperative day 12: hypotension and low cardiac output related to

- vasodilation (low systemic vascular resistance)
- depressed myocardial function
- increased capillary permeability

Adequate cardiac output as evidenced by

- systolic blood pressure > 90 mm Hg
- cardiac index > 2.5 liters/min/m$^2$
- urinary output > 20–30 ml/hour
- systemic vascular resistance > 800–1,200 dynes-sec/cm$^{-5}$
- full, strong peripheral pulses
- warm, dry, pink skin
- normal sensorium

The nurse will

- monitor heart rate and blood pressure every 30 min and as needed
- check hemodynamic profile every 2–4 hours
- monitor pulmonary artery end-diastolic and pulmonary capillary wedge pressures every 1–2 hours for volume status
- titrate vasopressor drips to keep
- systolic blood pressure > 90 mm Hg
- systemic vascular resistance > 800 dynes-sec/cm$^{-5}$
- cardiac index > 2.5 liters/min/m$^2$
- check urine output hourly
- administer volume expanders as ordered when volume depleted
- administer steroids as ordered; monitor for side-effects such as gastrointestinal irritation, hyperglycemia, hyponatremia or hyperkalemia

**Exhibit 5–1** Sample Form To Record Hemodynamic Profiles

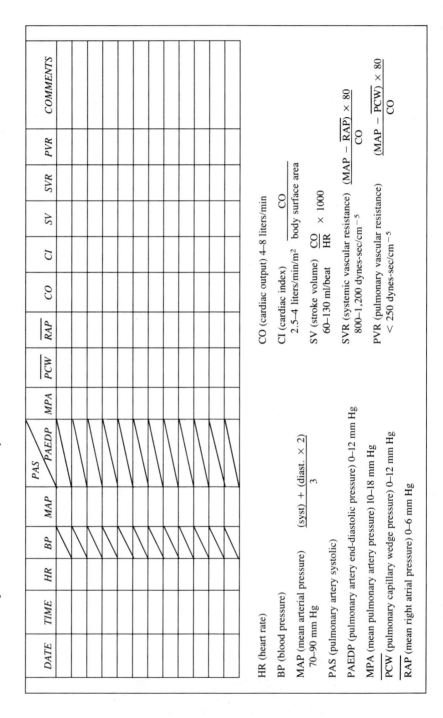

| DATE | TIME | HR | BP | MAP | PAS / PAEDP | MPA | $\overline{PCW}$ | $\overline{RAP}$ | CO | CI | SV | SVR | PVR | COMMENTS |
|------|------|----|----|-----|-------------|-----|------------------|------------------|----|----|----|-----|-----|----------|
| | | | | | | | | | | | | | | |
| | | | | | | | | | | | | | | |
| | | | | | | | | | | | | | | |
| | | | | | | | | | | | | | | |
| | | | | | | | | | | | | | | |
| | | | | | | | | | | | | | | |
| | | | | | | | | | | | | | | |
| | | | | | | | | | | | | | | |
| | | | | | | | | | | | | | | |
| | | | | | | | | | | | | | | |
| | | | | | | | | | | | | | | |
| | | | | | | | | | | | | | | |
| | | | | | | | | | | | | | | |

HR (heart rate)

BP (blood pressure)

MAP (mean arterial pressure)    $\dfrac{(\text{syst}) + (\text{diast.} \times 2)}{3}$
70–90 mm Hg

PAS (pulmonary artery systolic)

PAEDP (pulmonary artery end-diastolic pressure) 0–12 mm Hg

MPA (mean pulmonary artery pressure) 10–18 mm Hg

$\overline{PCW}$ (pulmonary capillary wedge pressure) 0–12 mm Hg

RAP (mean right atrial pressure) 0–6 mm Hg

CO (cardiac output) 4–8 liters/min

CI (cardiac index)    $\dfrac{CO}{\text{body surface area}}$
2.5–4 liters/min/m²

SV (stroke volume)    $\dfrac{CO}{HR} \times 1000$
60–130 ml/beat

SVR (systemic vascular resistance)    $\dfrac{(MAP - \overline{RAP}) \times 80}{CO}$
800–1,200 dynes-sec/cm⁻⁵

PVR (pulmonary vascular resistance)    $\dfrac{(MAP - \overline{PCW}) \times 80}{CO}$
< 250 dynes-sec/cm⁻⁵

**NOTES**

1. Vee Rice, "The Critical Continuum of Septic Shock," *Critical Care Nurse* 4 (September/October 1984):86–109.
2. Marguerite Rogers Kinney et al., *AACN's Clinical Reference for Critical Care Nursing* (New York: McGraw-Hill, 1981), 821–849.
3. W.R. McCabe, "Gram-Negative Bacteremia," *Diagnostic Medicine* (December 1983): 1–38.
4. M. Parker and J. Parrillo, "Septic Shock, Hemodynamics, and Pathogenesis," *Journal of the American Medical Association* 250 (1983): 3324–3327.
5. Beth Keely, "Septic Shock," *Critical Care Quarterly* 7 (March 1985): 59–67.
6. Rice, "The Critical Continuum."
7. Kinney et al., *AACN's Clinical Reference.*
8. Rice, "The Critical Continuum."
9. Anne Perry and Patricia Potter, *Shock* (St. Louis: C.V. Mosby, 1983).
10. Ibid.
11. Marilyn Roderick, *Infection Control in Critical Care* (Rockville, Md: Aspen Publishers, 1983), 87–107.
12. Kinney et al., *AACN's Clinical Reference.*
13. Perry and Potter, *Shock.*
14. Arthur Guyton, *Textbook of Medical Physiology,* 5th ed. (Philadelphia, W.B. Saunders, 1981).
15. Rice, "The Clinical Continuum."
16. G.T. Shires et al., "Changes in Red Blood Cell Transmembrane Potential, Electrolytes, and Energy Content in Septic Shock," *Journal of Trauma* 23 (1983): 769–774.
17. B.S. Kaufman, E.C. Rackow, and J.L. Faulk, "The Relationship between Oxygen Delivery and Consumption during Fluid Resuscitation of Hypovolemic and Septic Shock," *Chest* 85 (1984): 336–340.
18. Rice, "The Critical Continuum."
19. Ibid.

# Chapter 6

# Adult Respiratory Distress Syndrome

*Judy Dixon Fox, R.N., M.S.N.*

Adult respiratory distress syndrome (ARDS) is a pulmonary disorder known by many names: shock lung, white lung, adult hyaline membrane disease, and, more recently, noncardiogenic pulmonary edema. ARDS has often been reported in patients who have experienced trauma, with or without chest injury. In more recent years, however, it has been noted in a variety of conditions. Some of the conditions that may increase the risk of ARDS include embolism, obstetric complications, sepsis, burns, cardiopulmonary bypass, bacterial or interstitial pneumonias, and shock of any cause.

Although the mechanism of injury to the lungs that produces ARDS remains unclear in many conditions, the physiologic changes that occur and the resulting clinical presentations are very similar. The clinical presentation of ARDS includes

- interstitial and intra-alveolar edema
- increased vascular shunting
- decreased pulmonary compliance
- hypoxia

A mortality rate of greater than 50 percent has generally been associated with ARDS, but the overall mortality rate may range from 35 to 95 percent. There appears to be a relationship between the speed of clinical onset, severity of the disease course, and mortality rate. Those patients who develop clinical symptoms of ARDS soon after the original physical insult often have more severe cases, as well as much higher mortality rates.[1,2]

Mr. B, a 68-year-old man with a history of mild chronic obstructive pulmonary disease, had been sick at home for several days with increasing pulmonary congestion, a productive cough, and fever of 101°F. He came to the emergency department (ED) when his breathing difficulties increased. Clinical findings included a respiration rate of 44 breaths/ min, rales audible over the right lung field, and a cough that produced thick, yellow sputum. Radiologic examination indicated the presence of a right lower lobe infiltrate. A peripheral intravenous (IV) line was started with 5% dextrose .45 normal saline (D5½NS) infusing at 75 ml/ hour. A continuous aminophylline drip was initiated, and aerosol treat- ments of isoetharine (Bronchosol) in saline were given. Blood gas values revealed poor gas exchange with a $Pao_2$ of 55 mm Hg, a $Paco_2$ of 22 mm Hg, a pH of 7.48, and oxygen saturation of 82 percent. Mr. B was placed on a 40 percent oxygen mask and admitted to the intensive care unit (ICU). His condition was diagnosed as a bacterial pneumonia in the right lower lobe. Within 24 hours of admission, however, a secondary diagnosis of ARDS was made.

## HEMODYNAMIC MONITORING FOR THE ARDS PATIENT

The pathologic changes associated with ARDS that affect normal hemo- dynamics include a bilateral increase in cell membrane permeability, although the mechanisms that produce this alteration are not fully understood. Because of the increased permeability, fluid flows from the capillary into the interstitium and then into the alveolar sacs, where it causes a widespread pulmonary edema and increased vascular shunting. Under normal conditions, a small amount of blood may be shunted through the pulmonary capillary beds without making contact with ventilated alveoli; when the alveoli are filled with fluid, however, this shunting of unoxygenated blood into the systemic circulation increases and hypoxia results.[3-5]

The interstitial and intra-alveolar edema seen in the ARDS patient differs from the pulmonary edema that occurs in the patient with congestive heart failure. These differences include the pathophysiologic alterations that produce the edema, the composition of the fluid itself, and the changes in various hemo- dynamic parameters that result from the altered pulmonary state.

Three factors affect fluid flow across cellular membranes: (1) the capillary hydrostatic pressure, (2) protein osmotic pressures, and (3) the permeability of the capillary membrane. Increased alveolar fluid of a cardiac origin results from elevated intravascular hydrostatic and osmotic pressures that force fluid through the pulmonary vascular membrane into the interstitium and alveoli. These ele- vated pressures can be reflected by increases in pulmonary artery and pulmonary capillary wedge pressures. With no alteration in normal membrane permeability, large molecules cannot pass through the tight capillary linings. The edematous fluid, therefore, contains little or no cellular components or proteins.[6-9]

The fluid in the ARDS lung results from a change in the permeability of the cell wall, without elevations in hydrostatic or osmotic pressures. The patient with ARDS initially has no increase in pulmonary artery or pulmonary capillary wedge pressures, despite clinical evidence of pulmonary edema. Although pressures are not increased, the leaky capillary membranes allow larger molecules to enter the interstitium and alveoli. Therefore, the edematous fluid becomes exudate, containing such material as leukocytes, red blood cells, macrophages, and various protein material. The leakage of this fluid into the interstitium and alveoli produces pulmonary edema, increases shunting of unoxygenated blood into the systemic circulation, and destroys pulmonary surfactant. In turn, this decreases pulmonary compliance, which exacerbates the refractory hypoxia so characteristic of ARDS.[10–12]

Hypoxia itself can produce various hemodynamic changes. It can have a direct effect on the pulmonary vasculature, producing a pulmonary vasoconstriction. This effect can be monitored by the derived parameter of pulmonary vascular resistance, because vasoconstriction in the pulmonary beds is reflected in increases in the pulmonary vascular resistance.[13] As hypoxia worsens, the amount of oxygen available becomes inadequate to meet cellular demands. As cellular metabolism converts from an aerobic to an anaerobic process, shock develops, with further hemodynamic effects. Changes can be seen in those factors that determine cardiac output, such as heart rate, myocardial contractile force, and peripheral vasoconstriction. The cardiac output and systemic blood pressure can be monitored directly, while peripheral vasoconstriction can be monitored by means of the derived parameter of systemic vascular resistance. Derived parameters can be adjusted to a patient's body surface area to determine the cardiac index and to obtain a more accurate clinical assessment of the data.[14]

Another parameter now being used to monitor effective tissue oxygenation is mixed venous oxygen saturation ($Svo_2$). Researchers have developed fiberoptic pulmonary artery catheters that use the blood color spectrum to measure continuous $Svo_2$ at the bedside. Although normal values may vary somewhat from individual to individual, an $Svo_2$ of 75 percent is generally considered normal. This measurement provides much information on tissue oxygenation and the impact of the disease or its treatment.[15,16]

On arrival in the ICU, Mr. B was tachypneic and his pulmonary status was deteriorating rapidly. Rales were audible bilaterally, and he was becoming mentally disoriented to time and place. Further assessment revealed a heart rate of 128 beats/min, a respiration rate of 52 breaths/min, and a blood pressure of 80/40 mm Hg. Mr. B had required more supplemental oxygen, and his blood gas values while he was using a 50 percent oxygen mask were $Pao_2$, 34 mm Hg; $Paco_2$, 26 mm Hg; pH, 7.38; and oxygen saturation, 68 percent. Mr. B was intubated and breathing spontaneously on the ventilator at a rate of 32 breaths/min. Initial ventilatory settings were tidal volume, 1,000 ml; fraction of inspired oxygen ($Fio_2$), 50 percent; rate of mechanical ventilation (f) 8/ min. Blood gas values on these ventilator settings were $Pao_2$, 46 mm Hg; $Paco_2$, 17 mm Hg; pH, 7.49; and oxygen saturation 85 percent.

The appropriate antibiotics and an aminophylline drip that had been initiated in the ED was continued. A dopamine drip was connected in the ICU to improve blood pressure, and IV fluids were decreased to keep open rate. An arterial line was inserted for continuous monitoring of blood pressure and mean arterial pressure. A pulmonary artery catheter with an extra infusion port was also inserted; pressure waveforms from both the pulmonary artery and arterial lines were normal. Before insertion of the pulmonary artery catheter, the ventilator parameters were changed to improve oxygen delivery. After line insertion had been completed, a hemodynamic profile was done and blood gas values checked (Table 6–1). Radiologic examinations at this time revealed a bilateral infiltration process. The diagnosis of ARDS was made on the basis of radiologic findings and clinical presentations, including refractory hypoxia.

## MANAGEMENT OF HEMODYNAMIC PARAMETERS

The treatment of ARDS begins with the treatment of the primary condition; in Mr. B's case, it began with the initiation of antibiotic therapy. Other therapies used in the management of the ARDS patient are generally aimed at treating specific clinical problems as they develop.[1] One such problem is the alteration of normal blood gas values. Mr. B's blood gas values (see Table 6–1) evidenced hypoxia, despite high percentages of supplemental oxygen and ventilatory adjuncts, such as positive end expiratory pressure (PEEP). Interestingly, pH values are usually normal in the patient with ARDS. Hyperventilation, which decreases the $Paco_2$, is a compensatory mechanism used to control the acid-base balance. The pH is altered only after prolonged severe hypoxemia and shock, when changes in respiratory rates can no longer control the pH.[17–19]

Hypoxia can alter normal hemodynamics. Often, the therapies used to correct hypoxia alter hemodynamic values as well. Hypoxia-produced shock states may be evidenced by decreases in the cardiac output and mean arterial pressure, with increases in the systemic vascular resistance and pulmonary vascular resistance indexes. In order to improve his cardiac output and mean arterial pressure, Mr. B received a continuous infusion of dopamine. The dosage of dopamine was calculated according to his body weight and clinical response. Dopamine increases systemic vascular resistance and, through its inotropic properties, may increase

**Table 6–1** Mr. B: Hemodynamic and Ventilatory Parameters

| | Day 1 | Day 4 | Day 7 | Day 10 |
|---|---|---|---|---|
| **Hemodynamic Profile** | | | | |
| Heart rate | 102 beats/min | 150 beats/min | 139 beats/min | 130 beats/min |
| Blood pressure | 92/52 mm Hg | 126/48 mm Hg | 128/46 mm Hg | 98/42 mm Hg |
| Mean arterial pressure | 77 mm Hg | 75 mm Hg | 73 mm Hg | 60 mm Hg |
| Pulmonary artery pressure | 34/19 mm Hg | 52/30 mm Hg | 40/24 mm Hg | 36/20 mm Hg |
| Right atrial pressure | 8 mm Hg | 14 mm Hg | 14 mm Hg | 10 mm Hg |
| Pulmonary capillary wedge pressure | 13 mm Hg | 26 mm Hg | 22 mm Hg | 18 mm Hg |
| Cardiac output | 4.2 liters/min | 9.32 liters/min | 7.80 liters/min | 5.01 liters/min |
| Cardiac index | 2.1 liters/min/m$^2$ | 4.7 liters/min/m$^2$ | 3.9 liters/min/m$^2$ | 2.5 liters/min/m$^2$ |
| Systemic vascular resistance index | 1,906 dyne-sec/cm$^{-5}$ | 1,503 dyne-sec/cm$^{-5}$/m$^2$ | 1,202 dyne-sec/cm$^{-5}$/m$^2$ | 1,598 dyne-sec/cm$^{-5}$/m$^2$ |
| Pulmonary vascular resistance index | 406 dyne-sec/cm$^{-5}$ | 525 dyne-sec/cm$^{-5}$/m$^2$ | 594 dyne-sec/cm$^{-5}$/m$^2$ | 231 dyne-sec/cm$^{-5}$/m$^2$ |
| **Ventilatory Values** | | | | |
| Tidal volume | 1,000 ml | 1,000 ml | 1,000 ml | 1,000 ml |
| Rate of mechanical ventilation (f) | 8/min | 12/min | 12/min | 10/min |
| Fraction of inspired oxygen ($Fio_2$) | 70% | 50% | 70% | 90% |
| Positive end expiratory pressure (PEEP) | 6 cm $H_2O$ | 9 cm $H_2O$ | 12 cm $H_2O$ | 15 cm $H_2O$ |
| $Pao_2$ | 63 mm Hg | 65 mm Hg | 65 mm Hg | 58 mm Hg |
| $Paco_2$ | 31 mm Hg | 38 mm Hg | 27 mm Hg | 30 mm Hg |
| pH | 7.40 | 7.41 | 7.57 | 7.49 |
| Oxygen saturation | 91% | 98% | 94% | 91% |

myocardial contractile force and improve stroke volume.[20] Mr. B's blood pressure and mean arterial pressure improved after the administration of dopamine. The initial systemic vascular resistance index was calculated after the infusion of dopamine had begun, making it difficult to identify the extent to which the elevated systemic vascular resistance index was caused by shock and the extent to which it was caused by the drug.

The use of supplemental oxygen and bronchodilators (e.g., aminophylline) was an early attempt to improve oxygenation. Aminophylline, a xanthine derivative, is a commonly used bronchodilator that can be administered intravenously. Its primary effect is to dilate smooth muscle, thus enlarging the airway passages and improving air flow. Because this effect extends to the vascular system, it decreases the pulmonary vascular resistance index through dilation of the pulmonary vascular beds.[21] Hypoxia may increase the pulmonary vascular resistance, which decreases blood flow and oxygen transport; aminophylline therapy is often used to manage an elevated pulmonary vascular resistance and, thus, to improve oxygen delivery and transport.

Mechanical ventilation also produces hemodynamic changes. Positive pressure ventilation increases thoracic pressures on the vasculature, which decreases venous return. Alterations in venous return may be reflected in decreases in cardiac output and mean arterial pressure. Positive pressure ventilation also increases the central venous pressure (CVP), right atrial pressure, pulmonary artery pressure, and pulmonary capillary wedge pressure because of the combined effects of increased intrapleural and transmural pressures.[22–24]

The hemodynamic alterations that result from positive pressure ventilation are dependent on the amount of pressure delivered, especially when such adjuncts as PEEP are used. As the amount of PEEP increases, so does the impedance of venous return. This, of course, decreases cardiac output. Researchers are now demonstrating that other factors may also contribute to the decreased cardiac output. Studies have shown that PEEP can affect ventricular function and variables of stroke volume; for example, it may decrease ventricular distensibility, alter right and left transmural pressures, and increase pulmonary vascular resistance.[25] Mr. B demonstrated elevated pulmonary artery, right atrial, and pulmonary capillary wedge pressures while on mechanical ventilation and PEEP; however, his history of mild chronic obstructive pulmonary disease may have contributed to these elevations.

The management of pulmonary artery pressure and fluid status in the care of ARDS patients is controversial. Much of this controversy revolves around the selection of colloid or crystalloid solutions as fluid replacements. Those who advocate the use of colloids believe that osmotic solutions, such as albumin, pull fluid out of the interstitium and return it to the vascular beds, thus decreasing pulmonary edema. On the other side of this controversy are those who feel that the use of colloid and protein solutions increases pulmonary edema and damage because of the pathologic changes that occur in ARDS. As previously noted, the leaky capillary membranes seen in ARDS allow proteins to enter the edematous fluid; therefore, the use of crystalloids may dilute the protein-rich edematous fluid and decrease osmotic pressure. Increasingly, the choice of a colloid or crystalloid is determined by the individual patient's clinical progress and response to treatment.[26–28]

> On day 2 in the ICU, Mr. B was still having difficulty maintaining adequate oxygenation on the ventilator. A radiologic examination revealed bilateral infiltrates. Clinically, Mr. B had a sinus tachycardia of 140 to 210 beats/min. His blood pressure was stable on low-dose dopamine at 5 µg/kg/min. In the hope that a more isotonic solution would reduce the protein content of the edematous fluid, IV fluids were changed from D5½NS to 45% normal saline (½NS). Rales and rhonchi could be auscultated in lung fields bilaterally, and Mr. B continued to have a spontaneous respiration rate of 18 to 22 breaths/min. Blood gas values were determined frequently to monitor oxygenation, and ventilator settings were changed. In order to control all ventilatory parameters, a neuroblocking agent was needed. Therapy with pancuronium bromide (Pavulon) was initiated to stop all spontaneous respiratory efforts. In conjunction with the Pavulon, which has no sedative effects, IV diazepam (Valium) was routinely given. Once Pavulon had been given and paralysis was complete, it was no longer possible to assess changes in mental state adequately.
>
> Day 4 of Mr. B's hospitalization showed essentially no change in clinical or radiologic findings. He maintained a sinus tachycardia of 120 to 150 beats/min. Drug therapies continued to include a dopamine drip infused at 3 to 5 µg/kg/min, an aminophylline drip infused at 24 mg/ hour, and Pavulon given every 2 to 4 hours as needed. Valium continued to be given IV for its sedative effects during Pavulon therapy. Intermittent doses of furosemide (Lasix) were given to help control pulmonary edema. Hemodynamic and ventilatory parameters at this time are recorded in Table 6–1.
>
> Mr. B continued to have problems with hypoxia and pulmonary edema. Albumin was now being infused intermittently, in conjunction with the Lasix, in an attempt to manage the edema. Hemodynamic and ventilatory parameters on day 7 are shown in Table 6–1. There was some improvement in the pulmonary artery pressure after Mr. B had been given a total of 100 g albumin, although no change in the right atrial pressure was noted. Ventilatory status had deteriorated further, and increases in PEEP and supplemental oxygen were required to maintain marginal blood gas values.

**Table 6–2** Nursing Care Plan: ARDS

| Patient Problem | Patient Goals | Target Date | Nursing Actions |
|---|---|---|---|
| Alteration in gas exchange related to ARDS | The patient will have improved gas exchange as evidenced by<br><br>• blood gas values within normal limits;<br>  • $Pao_2$, 80–100 mm Hg<br>  • $Paco_2$, 35–45 mm Hg<br>  • pH, 7.35–7.45<br>  • oxygen saturation, 95%–100%<br>• pulmonary vascular resistance index within normal limits: 225–315 dyne-sec/cm$^{-5}$/m$^2$<br>• heart rate < 100 beats/min<br>• intact neurologic status when patient not receiving Pavulon | Day of admission | The nurse will<br><br>• maintain pulmonary toilet by<br>  • performing endotracheal suction every 2 hours and as needed, using sterile saline to liquefy secretions<br>  • preoxygenating with 100% $O_2$ while suctioning to prevent hypoxia<br>  • maintaining PEEP during suctioning procedure<br>• maintain positioning that will provide maximum tidal volume and decrease pooling of secretions:<br>  • side to side every 2 hours<br>  • elevation of head of bed 30°<br>• monitor blood gas values as ordered and notify physician of abnormalities<br>• monitor hemodynamic profile for increase in pulmonary vascular resistance index and any indication of impending shock:<br>  • elevation in systemic vascular resistance index and heart rate<br>  • decreases in blood pressure, mean arterial pressure, cardiac output, and cardiac index |

Potential shock related to

- increased cell membrane permeability
- altered hemodynamics
- fluid shifts

The patient will have no indication of shock as evidenced by

- hemodynamic values within normal limits:
  - mean arterial pressure, 70–90 mm Hg
  - pulmonary artery pressure, 10–25/0–12 mm Hg
  - pulmonary capillary wedge pressure, 0–12 mm Hg
  - cardiac output, 4–8 liters/min
  - cardiac index, 2.5–4 liters/min/m$^2$
  - systemic vascular resistance index, 1,970–2,390 dynes-sec/cm$^{-5}$/m$^2$
- heart rate < 100 beats/min
- urine output > 30 ml/hour
- blood gas values within normal limits
- clinical assessment
  - skin warm and dry
  - absence of cyanosis, neck vein distention, or peripheral vasoconstriction

Day of admission

The nurse will

- continually monitor and notify physician of abnormalities in heart rate, pulmonary artery pressure, mean arterial pressure, pulmonary capillary wedge pressure
- measure every 8 hours and as ordered cardiac output, cardiac index, systemic and pulmonary vascular resistance indexes; notify physician of abnormalities
- monitor and record as ordered blood gas values; notify physician of abnormalities
- notify physician of alterations in clinical findings
  - cyanosis
  - diaphoresis
  - increased pulmonary congestion
  - neck vein distention
  - cool skin with decreased capillary refill
- measure and record intake and output
- observe monitor for any cardiac dysrhythmias and intervene per protocol

**Table 6–2** continued

| Patient Problem | Patient Goals | Target Date | Nursing Actions |
|---|---|---|---|
| Potential hazards of immobility related to Pavulon therapy | The patient will not exhibit symptoms associated with immobility as evidenced by | Day of admission | The nurse will implement the following: |
| | • eyes/skin | | • eyes/skin |
| | • no drying or redness of sclera | | • administer artificial tears solution once Pavulon therapy started |
| | • pink skin without areas of redness, irritation, edema, or breakdown | | • use eye patches if excessive drying or redness develops |
| | • peripheral/vascular | | • place patient on foam |
| | • no edema | | • turn patient every 2 hours at a minimum |
| | • no localized heat or redness in legs | | • assess skin every 8 hours for irritation, redness, edema, or breakdown |
| | • gastrointestinal tract | | • keep skin clean and dry, avoid shearing force when turning patient |
| | • normally active bowel sounds in all quadrants | | • peripheral/vascular |
| | • bowel movement every 3–5 days | | • maintain passive range of motion exercises |
| | • no sign of abdominal distention or watery diarrhea | | • place pillow between knees to keep one leg from resting on the other leg |
| | • muscle tone | | • notify physician of any edema, redness, localized heat, or pain in legs |
| | • no sign of foot drop | | • muscle tone |
| | • no contractures | | • maintain passive range of motion exercises |
| | | | • place foot board on bed |

On day 10, IV fluids were being infused at a minimum rate. Lasix, albumin, and Pavulon therapies were being continued. The continuous infusion of aminophylline had been increased from 24 to 36 mg/hour. The hemodynamic profile at that time demonstrated an improvement in the pulmonary vascular resistance index and the pulmonary artery pressure, but the blood pressure, cardiac output, cardiac index, and mean arterial pressure were decreased (see Table 6–1). The dopamine drip was infusing at 9 $\mu$g/kg/min to maintain cardiac output and mean arterial pressure.

After 2 weeks of struggle to maintain oxygenation, Mr. B died. Death was attributed to ARDS secondary to bacterial pneumonia. At the time of his death, Mr. B was receiving aminophylline at 60 mg/hour and dopamine at varying rates to control blood pressure and mean arterial pressure. Ventilatory settings were tidal volume, 1,000 ml; $Fio_2$, 100 percent; f, 20/min; and PEEP, 15 cm $H_2O$. Pulmonary artery end-diastolic pressures were ranging 16 to 22 mm Hg, and the last reported blood gas values were $Pao_2$, 38 mm Hg; $Paco_2$, 52 mm Hg; pH, 7.22; and oxygen saturation, 61 percent.

Ultimately, the cause of an ARDS patient's death is hypoxia and its effects. The use of hemodynamic monitoring and interpretation of those parameters assist the clinician in providing more effective patient care. Still, ARDS is difficult to manage and, as in the case of Mr. B, is often fatal.

## NURSING CARE PLAN

A plan of care for Mr. B had been developed on his admission to the ICU (Table 6–2).

---

**NOTES**

1. Teresa Shafer, "Nursing Care of the Patient with ARDS," *Critical Care Nurse* 1 (March/April 1981): 34–43.

2. Stephen M. Ayres, "Mechanisms and Consequences of Pulmonary Edema: Cardiac Lung, Shock Lung, and Principles of Ventilatory Therapy in Adult Respiratory Distress Syndrome," *American Heart Journal* 82 (1982): 97–112.

3. Ibid.

4. Charles J. Carrico and Joel H. Horovitz, "Post Injury Acute Pulmonary Failure," in *Care of the Trauma Patient,* ed. G.T. Shires (New York: McGraw-Hill, 1979), 597–615.

5. Phillip C. Hopewell, "Adult Respiratory Distress Syndrome," *Basics of RD* 7 (1979), 1–6.

6. Ayres, "Mechanisms and Consequences of Pulmonary Edema."

7. Carrico and Horovitz, "Post Injury Acute Pulmonary Failure."

8. Hopewell, "Adult Respiratory Distress Syndrome."

9. Arthur C. Guyton, ed., *Textbook of Medical Physiology* (Philadelphia: W.B. Saunders, 1981).

10. Ayres, "Mechanisms and Consequences of Pulmonary Edema."

11. Carrico and Horovitz, "Post Injury Acute Pulmonary Failure."

12. Hopewell, "Adult Respiratory Distress Syndrome."

13. Frances Osgood et al., "Hemodynamic Monitoring in Respiratory Care," *Respiratory Care* 29 (1984): 25–34.

14. Donald D. Trunkey, George F. Shelton, and John A. Collins, "The Treatment of Shock," in *The Management of Trauma,* ed. George D. Zuidema, Robert B. Rutherford, and William T. Ballinger (Philadelphia: W.B. Saunders, 1979), 80–101.

15. Kathleen M. White, "Completing the Hemodynamic Picture: $SVO_2$," *Heart and Lung* 14 (1985): 272–280.

16. John C. McMichan, "Continuous Monitoring of Mixed Venous Oxygen Saturation: Theory Applied to Practice," in *Continuous Measurement of Blood Oxygen Saturation in the High Risk Patient,* ed. John F. Schweiss (San Diego: Beach International, 1983), 27–44.

17. Shafer, "Nursing Care of the Patient with ARDS."

18. Ayres, "Mechanisms and Consequences of Pulmonary Edema."

19. Hopewell, "Adult Respiratory Distress Syndrome."

20. Mary W. Falconer et al., *The Drug, The Nurse, The Patient* (Philadelphia: W.B. Saunders, 1978).

21. Ibid.

22. E.G. King, "Influence on Mechanical Ventilation and Pulmonary Disease on Pulmonary Artery Pressure Monitoring: Part Two," *CMA Journal* 121 (1979): 901–903.

23. Chuck Phillips, "Think Transmural," *Critical Care Nurse* 2 (1982): 36–44.

24. Michael A. Matthay, "Invasive Hemodynamic Monitoring in Acute Respiratory Failure," *Journal of Respiratory Disease* 2 (1982): 40–53.

25. Paul M. Dorinsky and Michael E. Whitcomb, "The Effects of PEEP on Cardiac Output," *Chest* (1983): 210–216.

26. Shafer, "Nursing Care of the Patient with ARDS."

27. Ayres, "Mechanisms and Consequences of Pulmonary Edema."

28. Carrico and Horovitz, "Post Injury Acute Pulmonary Failure."

# Chapter 7

# The Pediatric Patient

*Linda Gray Wofford, R.N., M.S.N., P.N.P.-C*

Hemodynamic monitoring has become increasingly accurate as advances in technology have made it easier to apply well-known hemodynamic principles. This is true for the pediatric patient as well as for the adult patient. It must be recognized, however, that children are not simply "little adults," they are unique in their physiologic and psychological needs. The physiologic differences between children and adults can be found in their body surface area, body water content, metabolic rate, cardiovascular system, and immunologic status.[1]

A child's body surface area is much greater in relation to his or her body mass than is an adult's body surface area.[2] The relatively larger body surface area provides a greater opportunity for heat and water dissipation through radiation, convection, and evaporation. Therefore, the child placed in a situation that increases heat and fluid loss, such as a radiant warmer that exposes the child to ambient air, must be carefully monitored. Small children also have higher total body water content and metabolic rates than do adults. The higher metabolic rates result in rapid depletion of body nutrients and rapid use of water reserves. These factors mandate meticulous attention to administered fluids—both oral and parenteral. The administration of fluids must be carefully calculated to achieve the proper balance between maintenance requirements, caloric needs, and patient output.

Because the child's cardiovascular system is much smaller than the adult's, smaller devices must be used for cannulation of the pediatric patient. Moreover, the pediatric cardiovascular system requires a highly sensitive monitoring mechanism, because even small quantitative changes in pressures are qualitatively significant.[3] The cardiac reserve in children is minute, and their small ventricles work at near capacity in producing stroke volume. The limited ventricular compliance of the child's heart, which is related to the greater proportion of non-contractile to contractile tissue,[4] makes it impossible for the child to increase cardiac output significantly by increasing stroke volume. Therefore, in the young

157

child, alteration in the heart rate is the major method to increase cardiac output and stroke volume. The child's variable and unpredictable response to endogenous catecholamines also distinguishes the pediatric patient from the adult patient. Contributing factors include an immature sympathetic nervous system and changing adrenergic receptors. This unpredictable response may include changes in vascular tone and inotropic states.[5]

Because hemodynamic monitoring usually involves invasive procedures, the immunologic status of the child must be considered. The health care team must be cognizant not only of the disease process for which the child is in the hospital, but also of the child's age-related susceptibility to infections. The immunoglobulins present in the newborn are different from those present in the 9-month-old infant. There is also a difference between the immune status of a 9-month-old infant and that of a 4-year-old preschooler.[6]

It is also important to remember that the pediatric patient's emotional and developmental needs are distinct from the adult's. Erikson's theory of development is useful in understanding these needs (Table 7–1). Because of these differences, both physical and psychological, the pediatric patient requires a unique nursing approach.

> Stacy, a 3-year-old white girl, was brought to the local emergency department with a 3-hour history of fever to 104.5°F, as well as chills, confusion, and a petechial rash. She was disoriented; had mottled, cyanotic skin; had a petechial rash over her entire body; and was cool to touch. Stacy's vital signs were temperature, 104.2°F; pulse 92; respiration rate, 36 breaths/min; and blood pressure 54/32 mm Hg. Her respirations were rapid and shallow with musical rales that could be auscultated bilaterally. Pulses were strong and equal, heart rate was rapid, but there was no murmur. The remaining physical findings were within normal limits, and her past medical and family history were unremarkable.
>
> Initially, a complete blood cell count with differential was ordered. The results demonstrated neutropenia. Cultures of blood, urine, and cerebrospinal fluid were obtained, followed by a chest roentgenogram, and metabolic studies. Broad-spectrum antibiotics were instituted to provide coverage against gram-negative and gram-positive bacteria. During the next 2 hours, Stacy's temperature continued to rise, her blood pressure continued to fall, and she was oliguric. Blood studies indicated a metabolic acidosis.

## USE OF HEMODYNAMIC MONITORING

The development of microtechniques in the late 1960s allowed more effective hemodynamic monitoring of critically ill children. In 1980, Finer described

**Table 7-1** Developmental and Emotional Needs of the Pediatric Patient

| Age Group Characteristics | Identified Parental Considerations | Nursing Interventions |
|---|---|---|
| *Infants (birth to 12 months)* | Bonding | Recognize identifiable changes in status |
| Developing sense of trust versus mistrust | Need encouragement to do "passive physiotherapy" (range of motion, stroking) | Adhere to strict handwashing and limitation of visitors |
| Not able to provide self-care | Need encouragement to do mothering tasks: feeding, touching, holding | Converse in a quiet, unabrupt manner |
| Requires expert respiratory management | | Encourage parents to do non-nursing aspects of care |
| Requires strict adherence to infection control | | Act as surrogate in absence of parents |
| Needs stimulation through sight and sound | | Provide mobiles to look at and toys to hold |
| Requires active play with toys | | |
| | | |
| *Toddler (ages 1 to 3 years)* | Need encouragement to provide comfort measures and communication | Encourage parental participation through example |
| Prime concern: sense of autonomy and fear of separation | Need encouragement in holding child at bedside | Offer explanations of thoughts child must feel, but cannot express, i.e., pain, Mommy not here |
| Is a dependent person, but has own mind and will | Need encouragement to participate in non-nursing aspects of care | Avoid participation in painful procedures: instead, offer comfort afterward by holding, stroking |
| Begins speech, albeit limited in use and vocabulary | | Use sedation and restraints only as necessary for safety |
| Concerned about integrity | | Demonstrate procedures and/or illness by dressing up toys, dolls, using puppets (child life worker) |
| Protects self from environment through avoidance, escape, and denial | | Hold, stroke, spend time with child, especially at bedtime if parents absent |
| Requires active play | | |
| Regards parents as most significant persons | | |
| Becomes especially lonely at bedtime | | |
| | | |
| *Pre-School (ages 3 to 6)* | Encourage participation in offering explanations of procedures and events, | Demonstrate and discuss procedures using understandable adult vocabulary |
| Wants to maintain acquired skills of doing for self; immobility frightening | | |

**Table 7-1** continued

| Age Group Characteristics | Identified Parental Considerations | Nursing Interventions |
|---|---|---|
| Has vivid imagination and sense of initiative | based on established trust with child | Allow child to participate in acquired tasks |
| Is acquiring language through limited use of words | Encourage reading, game playing, activities based on limits of child's illness | Permit questions: understand denial through withdrawal |
| Imitates adult behavior with potential accompanying sense of guilt | Need encouragement to participate in non-nursing aspects of care | Dress up toys for child to demonstrate fears (child life worker) |
| Develops concept of self and non-self by exploring environment and body and by questioning | Encourage holding, stroking, communication | Use restraints only as necessary for safety: sedation for pain and to allay fear of immobility |
| Regards family members as significant persons | | Encourage emotional ties with home by encouraging parents to bring in a child's favorite toys, games, pictures of pets and siblings, tape recordings |
| *School Age (ages 6 to 12)* | | |
| Needs recognition of accomplishment; has strong sense of duty | Encourage reading, game playing, activities based on limits of child's illness | Ascertain child's level of understanding to identify and correct misconceptions and offer explanations at his level |
| Inferiority through unattainable achievement can deplete sense of identity | Need encouragement to provide comfort measures; can act as go-between in communication for explanations and reinforcement | Permit child participation in progressive self-care |
| Capable of verbalizing pain | | Understand and offer comfort for parental separation |
| May demand an overabundance of love and attention from mother and regress | Encourage holding, stroking | Be aware of verbal, nonverbal indication of pain and sedate accordingly |
| Requires that limits be set to foster a sense of security | Need encouragement to participate in non-nursing aspects of care | Use child life worker for play therapy |
| Regards school and related events as main focus of significant persons | Assist in reality orientation with news of school and home | |
| *Puberty Adolescence (ages 12 to 19 years)* | | |
| Seeking identity, independence, and clarification of role in society after separation from family | Need to understand potential for regression | Treat as adult based on level of psychological adjustment |
| | Need encouragement to promote awareness of disease and prognosis | Recognize and foster independence through participation in care |
| Especially vulnerable to depersonalization and regression | Encourage treating adolescent as an adult | Set limits, but encourage decision making of adolescent in planning of care |
| Loss of body control destroys sense of pride | Can bring news of peer group and home events | |

Attempting to identify own sense of
belonging, self-esteem
Concerned with body image change through
surgery or illness
Regards peer group as significant persons

Include peers in visiting policies, since
relationships are moving away from family
Use music as a comfort measure

*Source:* Reprinted from *Pediatric Clinics of North America*, Vol. 27, No. 3, pp. 628–629, with permission of W.B. Saunders Company, © 1980.

several sophisticated tools capable of continuous monitoring.[7] When he compared transcutaneous oxygen monitoring by means of a heated Clark skin electrode to continuous oxygen monitoring by means of an intra-arterial catheter with a polygraphic electrode, he found a high correlation between the two methods (r = 0.79 and 0.71). (He cautioned practitioners that 12 percent of the polygraphic electrodes failed to activate, however.) Finer also reported that the transcutaneous oxygen electrodes provide an accurate, noninvasive method to monitor peripheral oxygen delivery.

Other tools available for continuous monitoring of intravascular oxygen saturation are the ear oximeter and the double lumen fiberoptic catheter. To date, both these tools are large and, therefore, difficult to use in pediatric patients. The ear oximeter must be held in place for infants and small children, while the fiberoptic catheter can be used only for older children. Similarly, a device used to measure carbon dioxide by means of an in-dwelling catheter attached to a mass spectrometer has not yet been perfected for use in infants and small children. Carbon dioxide can be monitored transcutaneously by means of pH-sensitive glass electrodes placed on the child's skin or heated infrared transducers applied to an area of stripped epidermis, however. Finer reports that the nonheated electrodes responded much more slowly, were less accurate, and required greater operator time for calibration and regulation than did the heated transducers.[8]

Arterial blood pressure in children is usually monitored by means of a series of cannulas, tubings, stopcocks, and transducers. Successful monitoring of arterial blood pressure with transducers produces an arterial waveform in which the systolic pressure and diastolic pressure are clearly indicated. The selection of the site for arterial cannulation is determined by the stability of the artery and the availability of collateral circulation. The radial artery offers the best collateral circulation and the least stability. In contrast, the femoral artery provides exceptional stability and limited collateral circulation.

Venous pressure is typically monitored with a central venous pressure (CVP) line that is inserted percutaneously or via a cutdown into the superior vena cava. Once the CVP line has been correctly positioned, it is useful in obtaining direct information about venous return, blood volume, and right ventricular function, as well as indirect information about the pulmonary vascular system. The normal pediatric CVP values are 1 to 7 mm Hg[9] or 6 to 15 cm $H_2O$.[10] Perhaps the single most important factor in monitoring CVP is the consistency of the technique. In addition to their usefulness in hemodynamic monitoring, CVP lines are useful in obtaining blood samples and infusing vasoactive drugs and hypertonic solutions.

The mean pulmonary capillary wedge pressure in children is normally 5 to 12 mm Hg.[11] This pressure is monitored by a floating balloon-tipped catheter that is inserted into the venous system and threaded into the pulmonary circulation. Because there is a risk of catheter migration, which can result in arrhythmias or pulmonary infarction, the waveform should be monitored continuously.

Because of improved technology, the health care professional is now able to monitor pulmonary and left ventricular filling pressures. The development of the flow-directed balloon-tipped Swan-Ganz catheter has allowed more accurate hemodynamic monitoring of intracardiac and pulmonary pressures in the intensive care unit. This catheter can be used to assess right ventricular function, flow and resistance in the pulmonary vascular bed, left ventricular function, and cardiac output. Placement of the Swan-Ganz catheter must be continuously monitored by observation of the pressure tracing to ensure that the catheter does not become wedged into the smaller pulmonary artery branches, where it could cause a pulmonary infarction. Therefore, in order to minimize the complications associated with monitoring pulmonary and left ventricular filling pressures, the health care team must be familiar with the hemodynamic parameters for pediatric and adult patients (Table 7–2).

With a working diagnosis of septic shock, Stacy was admitted directly to the intensive care unit. In order to maintain adequate ventilation, humidified oxygen was administered by nasal cannula. An arterial line was established to monitor blood gas levels, and a Swan-Ganz catheter was inserted to determine venous return, blood volume, cardiac output, and pulmonary vascular flow and resistance. Table 7–3 contains Stacy's hemodynamic parameters at this time. In order to stabilize her CVP, reverse hypovolemia, and increase urine output, Stacy was given

**Table 7–2** Comparison of Pediatric and Adult Hemodynamic Parameters

|  | Pediatric | Adult |
|---|---|---|
| *Pressure norms:* | | |
| CVP mean | 1–7 mm Hg | 4–8 mm Hg |
| PCWP mean | 6–12 mm Hg | 10–12 mm Hg |
| PAP mean | 10–12 mm Hg | 8–12 mm Hg |
| *Cardiac catheterization norms:* | | |
| RA mean | 2–6 mm Hg | 4–8 mm Hg |
| PA mean | 10–16 mm Hg | 10–12 mm Hg |
| LA mean | 5–10 mm Hg | 8–12 mm Hg |
| LV phasic pressure | 90–110/6–12 mm Hg | 90–140/4–12 mm Hg |

*Note:* CVP, central venous pressure; PCWP, pulmonary capillary wedge pressure; PAP, pulmonary artery pressure; RA, right atrial; PA, pulmonary artery; LA, left atrial; LV, left ventricle.

*Source:* Adapted with permission of Elsevier Science Publishing Co., Inc. from *Pediatric Cardiology* by C.L. Anthony, R.G. Arnon, and C.W. Fitch. Copyright © 1979 by Medical Examination Publishing Company, Inc.

a carefully monitored, large volume of isotonic electrolyte solution. Following these interventions, isoproterenol was administered to decrease her peripheral vascular resistance.

Within 3 hours, Stacy was normotensive and had an adequate urine output. Furthermore, all intracardiac and pulmonary pressures were within normal limits. She continued to receive carefully monitored parenteral fluids and broad-spectrum antibiotics. The antibiotic coverage was altered appropriately when the blood cultures showed that *Escherichia coli* was the causative organism of Stacy's bacteremia. As her condition stabilized and improved, Stacy's monitors were removed, and she was transferred from the intensive care unit to the general pediatric unit (see Table 7–3). Once on the pediatric unit, Stacy completed her antibiotic course. When fully recovered, she went home.

The successful use of hemodynamic monitoring in the pediatric patient is a careful blending of complex technical skills and applied knowledge of a child's growth and development. Most of the hemodynamic principles are the same for adults and children, but the application of those principles to the special people called children requires nursing care that meshes the science and art of the nursing profession.

## NURSING DIAGNOSIS AND CARE PLAN

A portion of the nursing care plan written for Stacy is shown in Table 7–4.

---

**Table 7–3** Stacy: Hemodynamic Parameters

|  | Line Insertion (mm Hg) | Line Removal (mm Hg) |
| --- | --- | --- |
| Central venous pressure (mean) | 1 | 5 |
| Pulmonary artery wedge pressure (mean) | 8 | 9 |
| Right atrial pressure (mean) | 3 | 4 |
| Pulmonary artery pressure (mean) | 10 | 12 |
| Left atrial pressure (mean) | 10 | 7 |
| Blood pressure | 80/8 | 92/10 |

**Table 7–4** Nursing Care Plan: The Pediatric Patient

| Patient Problem | Patient Goals | Nursing Actions |
|---|---|---|
| Actual infection | The patient will be free of signs and symptoms of infection as evidenced by | The nurse will |
| | • temperature <38°C for >36 hours | • observe and document vital signs, electrocardiogram |
| | • skin pink and warm; not flushed or clammy | • set bedside alarms |
| | • hemodynamic parameters within normal limits | • record cuff blood pressure every shift |
| |   • central venous pressure, 1–7 mm Hg | • record urine output every hour |
| |   • pulmonary capillary wedge pressure, 6–12 mm Hg | • obtain appropriate cultures if temperature spikes and notify physician |
| |   • pulmonary artery pressure, 10–20 mm Hg | • give fluids and/or vasodilators to keep hemodynamic parameters within desired limits |
| | • adequate urine output for age and weight, 2–3 ml/kg/hour | • administer antibiotics as ordered: separate β-lactam drugs and aminoglycosides by at least 1 hour; monitor potassium and administer supplements as ordered |
| | • mental status within normal limits | • prevent nosocomial infection by promoting good handwashing of all contacts and double preparing all venipuncture sites, tubing, stopcock, and cannula junctions |
| | • all cultures negative | • obtain appropriate drug levels to prevent toxic reactions and inadequate coverage |
| | • drug levels within therapeutic ranges | |
| Impaired gas exchange related to alteration of microcirculation by gram-negative endotoxin | The patient will demonstrate return of normal gas exchange as evidenced by | The nurse will |
| | • normal laboratory values | • administer oxygen to saturate available hemoglobin |
| |   • electrolytes | • administer large volumes of fluids to maintain adequate blood flow and pressor |
| |   • hemoglobin saturation | |

Actual self-esteem disturbance related to restrictive environment of pediatric intensive care unit

- arterial blood gases
- pressure tracings
- vascular resistance
- return to previous energy level
- skin pink and warm
- return to normal pulmonary function

The patient will demonstrate return of appropriate self-esteem as evidenced by

- making choices for himself/herself when offered
- building trusting relationships with staff, who are honest with patient about all procedures
- accepting procedures as necessary
- maintaining positive relationships with significant others
- showing or expressing pride in accomplishments during hospitalization

agents to restore normal vascular resistance

- monitor blood gas levels and pressure tracings
- limit the patient's activities to conserve energy
- reinforce the patient's orientation to person, place, and time
- evaluate the hypoxemia and acidosis
- assess for hemorrhage, atelectasis, edema, and capillary thrombi

The nurse will

- encourage autonomy by creating choices for the patient
- explain all procedures in honest language that is appropriate for cognitive level
- include significant others in patient's care to enhance personal security
- avoid activities and attitudes that foster shame and doubt

## NOTES

1. M.F. Hazinski, *Nursing Care of the Critically Ill Child* (St. Louis: C.V. Mosby, 1984), 648–737.
2. Ibid.
3. Ibid.
4. A. Zaritsky and B. Chernow, "Use of Catecholamines in Pediatrics," *Journal of Pediatrics* 105 (1984): 341–347.
5. Ibid.
6. S.R. Mott, N.F. Fazekas, and S.R. James, *Nursing Care of Children and Families: A Holistic Approach* (Menlo Park, Calif.: Addison-Wesley, 1985), 192, 258, 1016–1017.
7. N.N. Finer, "Newer Trends in Continuous Monitoring of Critically Ill Infants and Children," *Pediatric Clinics of North America* 27 (1980): 553–566, (1980).
8. Ibid.
9. C.L. Anthony, R.G. Arnon, and C.W. Fitch, *Pediatric Cardiology* (Garden City, N.Y.: Medical Examination Publishing, 1979).
10. S.A. Cohen, *Pediatric Emergency Management* (Bowie, Md: Prentice-Hall Publishing and Communications, 1982), 14.
11. G.W. Guido, "Instrumentation," in *Pediatric Critical Care Nursing,* ed. K.W. Vestal (New York: John Wiley & Sons, 1981), 158–186.

## REFERENCES

Brantigan, C.O. "Hemodynamic Monitoring: Interpreting Values." *American Journal of Nursing* 82 (1982): 86–89.

Hedges, J.R. "Preload and Afterload Revisited." *Journal of Emergency Nursing* 9 (1983): 262–267.

Hoekelman, R.A., Blatman, S., Brunell, P.A., Friedman, S.B., and Seidel, H.M. *Principles of Pediatrics: Health Care of the Young.* New York: McGraw-Hill, 1978.

Hurst, J.M. "Invasive Hemodynamic Monitoring: An Overview." *Journal of Emergency Nursing* 10 (1984): 11–22.

Norris, D.L., and Klein, L.A. "What All Those Pressure Readings Mean . . . and Why." *RN* 44 (1981): 35–42.

Perkin, R.M., and Levin, D.L. "Shock in the Pediatric Patient. Part I." *Journal of Pediatrics* 101 (1982): 163–169.

Perkin, R.M., Levin, D.L., Webb, R., Aquino, A., and Reedy, J. "Dobutamine: A Hemodynamic Evaluation in Children with Shock." *Journal of Pediatrics* 100 (1982): 977–983.

# Cardiac Surgery Following Acute Myocardial Infarction

*Jeannie Tharpe Sizemore, R.N., M.S.N.*

The care of patients who have experienced acute myocardial infarction (AMI) has become increasingly more aggressive since the development of coronary care units in 1960. Continuous electrocardiograms (ECGs) in the coronary care unit facilitated the identification and treatment of life-threatening dysrhythmias and led to a decreased mortality rate in this population. Prophylactic use of drugs to suppress ventricular ectopy further improved mortality statistics during this period.

Since then, various medical interventions have been pursued to protect ischemic myocardium. Among these was the administration of β-blockers to decrease the level of circulating catecholamines, which is elevated in AMI patients secondary to compensatory mechanisms. These drugs helped improve the oxygen supply:demand ratio by decreasing heart rate and contractility. It was postulated that, as oxygen demand decreased, ischemic zones of the infarcted myocardium would be allowed to regain their function. Although the β-blockers were of some benefit to the AMI patient, they were not as effective as had been hoped in protecting ischemic tissue during the acute phase of myocardial infarction.[1]

Another technique used to stabilize the ischemic myocardium was a glucose-insulin-potassium (GIK) infusion. In the process of AMI, coronary artery occlusion interrupts the aerobic metabolic pathways. GIK infusions were thought to improve anaerobic glycolysis by providing a ready fuel supply in the form of glucose.[2] The combination of glucose and insulin was also thought to facilitate more normal ionic gradients by promoting potassium entry into the cell. As ionic gradients were stabilized, it was postulated that dysrhythmias would decrease although actual studies on the clinical effects of GIK are not conclusive.

Unlike β-blockers and GIK infusions, which affect only one side of the myocardial oxygen supply:demand ratio, intra-aortic balloon pumping affects both sides; it improves oxygen supply and reduces oxygen demand. These dual effects were thought to improve myocardial efficiency.[3] Inflation of the balloon during diastole increases coronary artery blood flow; deflation before systole reduces the aortic blood pressure, thereby reducing afterload. Intra-aortic balloon pumping is used with varying degrees of enthusiasm in different institutions to stabilize the AMI patient.

Although experimental studies of each of these interventions had been promising, the results of their use in AMI patients were somewhat disappointing. In an effort to intervene in the cause of the AMI, rather than in the results, Gruntzig, Zeitler, and Schoop developed percutaneous transluminal coronary angioplasty (PTCA).[4] In this procedure, a ballooned catheter is advanced past the coronary lesion. The balloon is then inflated with a controlled inflation device for 3 to 5 seconds, dilating the occluded coronary artery. By 1979, Gruntzig, Senning, and Siegenthaler had performed 50 procedures with a success rate of 66 percent.[5] The success rate of PTCA, as well as the complication rate, seems to be related to the experience of the practitioners—with more experience, the success rate increases, and the complication rate decreases.[6]

Another procedure that has gained popularity recently is the infusion of streptokinase to dissolve clots that have formed in the coronary artery. This intervention, like PTCA, is intended to interrupt the causative factor in the evolving AMI. The disruption of the coronary thrombosis by streptokinase limits the lesion size in many cases, which improves left ventricular performance.[7,8] Although many physicians administer streptokinase directly into the coronary artery, promising results of peripheral intravenous administration of the drug suggest that this procedure may be safe and useful for patients who experience AMI in outlying hospitals.[9,10]

Many studies show that emergency coronary artery reconstruction can improve left ventricular performance and reduce ischemic pain by restoring blood flow to the ischemic myocardium.[11,12] The surgical mortality of surgery for acute evolving transmural myocardial infarction is reported by some to be approximately 4 percent if the operation is performed in the first 6 to 8 hours after the onset of pain.[13] Other groups report a 1.76 percent in-house mortality for patients who undergo surgery within the first 6 hours.[14,15] These statistics compare to a 11.5 percent mortality rate for AMI patients managed with conventional therapy.[16]

Clearly, care of the AMI patient has become more invasive and aggressive since the 1960s. Current hemodynamic monitoring techniques provide invaluable information for the care of these acutely ill patients. Along with hemodynamic information, echocardiography and radionuclide scanning provides physiologic measurements that are useful in the evaluation of each form of therapy. Although the method chosen for myocardial preservation varies from physician to physician, each procedure has some advantages and some disadvantages. Future research will, no doubt, help define specific patient populations who will benefit from each method of treatment.

Mr. S, a 52-year-old man, went to the emergency department because, for 1½ hours, he had felt a crushing chest pain that extended to both arms. His condition was diagnosed as acute myocardial infarction. He was treated with streptokinase by infusion and, subsequently, coronary artery bypass surgery.

## HEMODYNAMIC MONITORING IN THE AMI PATIENT AFTER SURGERY

The postoperative care of the cardiac surgical patient is a challenging and rewarding experience. Because of dramatic changes in hemodynamics following surgery, the immediate postoperative period is critical. After the initial few hours in which the patient requires much care and attention, there is a recuperative period in which tubes and devices are gradually discontinued and the patient begins an active rehabilitation process.

### Myocardial Preservation

Cardiac surgical patients are unique in many ways. The procedures used during surgery to preserve myocardium not only decrease the temperature of the heart, but also produce systemic hypothermia. Thus, in the early postoperative period, the patients generally have an elevated systemic vascular resistance as a result of vasoconstriction. This vasoconstriction is usually temporary and can be managed easily with vasodilator therapy until the patient has warmed to a more normal temperature. In some patients, however, measures to reduce afterload must be continued after warming.

Cooling the heart also depresses the sinus node function. Therefore, until the patient's temperature has returned to normal, atrial pacing may be necessary to ensure adequate cardiac output. Atrial pacing is preferred to ventricular pacing, because it produces a more normal sequence of events. If temporary atrial pacing wires are not available, ventricular pacing may be necessary. In this case, the ventricular rate may need to be somewhat higher to compensate for the lack of atrial input.

Ventricular irritability caused by hypothermia may produce ventricular ectopy and fibrillation. Lidocaine infusions may be helpful in reducing this risk, but the most effective treatment is rewarming. This is most frequently accomplished by cardiopulmonary bypass before the patient's return to the postoperative unit. For the rare patient who returns to the postoperative unit quite cold, it is critical to use warming blankets, heat lamps, or blood warmers to return the patient slowly to a normothermic state.

Hypothermia also decreases the ability of the blood to clot. Every effort should be made to return the patient to a normal temperature before weaning from cardiopulmonary bypass so that an assessment of bleeding can be made.

## Cardiopulmonary Bypass

While the surgery is being performed, cardiopulmonary bypass produces a simulated cardiac output. The priming solution used for bypass varies from institution to institution, but it is generally a solution that contains saline, blood or colloids, and heparin for anticoagulation. In addition, mannitol or furosemide (Lasix) can be added to stimulate some diuresis following the procedure, allowing the hematocrit to return to a more normal level. Because of the hemodilution, it is generally not necessary to give blood to optimize preload in the early postoperative period unless the hematocit is less than 30 percent.

The combination of cell destruction from cardiopulmonary bypass, heparinization, and hypothermia produces a transient anticoagulation that can cause bleeding problems. Red blood cell destruction is often evidenced by hemolyzed blood samples and hematuria. Although not generally severe, this condition should be monitored. Some physicians prefer to keep the patient's urine output high to prevent any renal damage as a result of the stasis of red blood cells. If the patient continues bleeding, fresh-frozen plasma is given to replenish other clotting factors.

After the surgical procedure, protamine is given according to the results of the activated clotting time determination. It is important to remember that this is a nonspecific clotting test and cannot be used to differentiate between inadequate heparin reversal and other clotting problems. If the activated clotting time remains elevated after adequate protamine administration, other causes of bleeding must be investigated and treated.

## Assessment of Cardiac Output

A systematic approach is required for the assessment of cardiac output in the early postoperative period. Because of the hypothermia, the patient's heart rate is rarely elevated above normal levels. Bradycardias can be managed easily by atrial or ventricular pacing. Interventions to manage bradycardias should be made before any attempt is made to optimize preload, afterload, or contractility.

Fluid shifts in the early postoperative period require constant attention in the assessment of preload. It may be necessary to administer additional fluids to optimize preload. Usually, fluid replacement includes packed red blood cells, albumin, or other volume expanders. Whole blood is rarely used because of the risk of hepatitis associated with its use. The left atrial or pulmonary capillary wedge pressure is generally maintained at approximately 6 to 10 mm Hg. Patients with mitral valve disease or long-standing cardiac failure generally require a higher filling pressure.

Other factors that influence preload must be considered in assessing the patient's status. Volume-cycled ventilators elevate pulmonary artery end-diastolic pressure and left atrial pressure by increasing intrathoracic pressure. The patient should not be taken off the ventilator for measurements of left atrial or pulmonary capillary wedge pressure, as this may induce hypoxemia and elevate pulmonary vascular resistance. The changes in pressure caused by mechanical ventilation should be evaluated by the nurse when limits/ranges for cardiopulmonary measurements are ordered by the physician. As the patient is weaned from the ventilator and intrathoracic pressures return to normal, an assessment of preload may indicate the need for additional fluids at this time.

Following optimization of heart rate and preload, afterload should be evaluated by calculating the systemic vascular resistance. If it is elevated, vasodilators should be administered carefully. Many surgical patients respond well to very low doses of such drugs as nitroprusside or nitroglycerine. Some vasodilator drugs affect both venous and arterial vascular beds, and a constant assessment of preload must accompany the administration of the drugs. If the systemic vascular resistance is elevated as a result of systemic hypothermia, it is usually necessary to reduce the dosage as the patient warms.

After all the other elements of cardiac output have been assessed, contractility should be evaluated. If the cardiac index is low despite optimization of heart rate, preload, and afterload, the patient may need positive inotropic support. Changes in contractility should be made only when absolutely necessary, because they increase oxygen consumption significantly. Furthermore, the administration of drugs that increase contractility when the patient is hypovolemic can cause a decrease in renal function by shunting blood away from the renal system.

## GOALS AND MANAGEMENT

The ultimate goal in the treatment of Mr. S was to salvage as much myocardial muscle mass as possible. His treatment began with an infusion of streptokinase to allow for reperfusion of the coronary artery. Following the infusion, coronary artery bypass surgery corrected the residual coronary artery stenosis.

Mr. S's vital signs on admission to the postoperative unit were blood pressure, 172/110; sinus tachycardia, 120 beats/min; and respiration rate, 20 breaths/min. The ECG revealed Q waves in leads $V_1$ through $V_3$ and a 2-mm ST depression in leads II, III, and aVF. Mr. S was given sublingual nitroglycerine and oxygen at 2 liters/min, which eased his chest discomfort. The chest pain recurred after 25 minutes, at which time he was given sublingual nifedipine (Procardia), 10 mg; a lidocaine infusion was started at 30 μg/kg/min for prophylaxis against ventricular ectopy during reperfusion. He was seen by the cardiologist, who diagnosed his condition as an acute anterior myocardial infarction. Because Mr. S's condition was diagnosed within 6 hours after the onset of chest pain, the cardiologist recommended immediate streptokinase infusion to salvage myocardial muscle and improve left ventricular performance.

Mr. S was taken to the catheterization laboratory, where he was given 250,000 units streptokinase into the left main coronary artery. At 15 minutes after the streptokinase infusion, the recannulization of the left anterior descending coronary artery revealed a 90 percent residual stenosis, at midsegment (Table 8–1). Mr. S's comfort increased and chest pain diminished as the left anterior descending coronary artery opened. He experienced a short run of ventricular tachycardia at the time of recannulization, which resolved spontaneously. ST segments returned to baseline at this time.

The Swan-Ganz catheter and sheath were left in place after catheterization because of the possibility of bleeding as a result of the streptokinase. An infusion of heparin was started, and dipyridamole

**Table 8–1** Mr. S: Cardiac Catheterization Data

| Hemodynamics | Left Ventricular Angiogram |
|---|---|
| Pulmonary artery pressure, 22/15 (17) mm Hg | Left ventricular size normal—anterolateral and septal akinesis |
| Pulmonary capillary wedge pressure, 7 mm Hg | |
| Left ventricle, 82/10/12 mm Hg | |
| Cardiac index, 1.94 liters/min/m$^2$ | |
| Aortic blood pressure 82/60 (68) | |
| Left main coronary artery | 20%–30% stenosis |
| Left anterior descending artery | 30% proximal stenosis with complete occlusion at midsegment; 90% residual stenosis poststreptokinase |
| Left circumflex | Nondominant with 10% stenosis between marginal$_1$ and marginal$_2$ |
| Marginal$_1$ | 70% proximal stenosis |
| Marginal$_2$ | 70% ostial stenosis |
| Right coronary artery | Dominant with diffuse 30% midsegment stenosis; other right coronary artery branches normal |

(Persantine) administered p.o. to maintain patency of the coronary arteries. Isosorbide dinitrate (Isordil), nitroglycerine (Nitrol) ointment, and nifedipine (Procardia) were also started at this time for reduction of afterload and dilation of the coronary arteries. Lidocaine infusion was continued at 30 μg/kg/min. Mr. S's vital signs and hemodynamic profile remained stable postcatheterization with a cardiac index 2.8 liters/min/m$^2$ (Table 8–2).

The next morning, the heparin drip was temporarily interrupted for 2 hours before the Swan-Ganz catheter and groin sheath were removed. Pressure was held at the site for 30 minutes after the devices were removed to control bleeding; a sandbag was placed over the site for 4 additional hours to provide hemostasis. Mr. S continued to progress well without chest pain. The partial thromboplastin time was maintained at twice the control by adjustments in the heparin dosage.

Mr. S's catheterization results were discussed with the cardiac surgeons. It was decided that, because of the severity of his residual stenosis, the best approach to his care would be coronary artery bypass grafting. After a discussion with his physicians and family, Mr. S agreed to proceed with the surgery, which was planned for 1 week after his myocardial infarction.

Extensive preoperative instructions were given to Mr. S and his family. They were taken on a tour of the intensive care unit, met the nurse who would care for him, and talked with patients in the unit. A preoperative nursing assessment was completed for planning care.

Mr. S underwent surgery for saphenous vein bypass grafts to the left anterior descending, diagonal, and second marginal arteries. He was

**Table 8–2** Mr. S: Post–Cardiac Catheterization Hemodynamic Profile

| Parameter | Patient | Normal |
|---|---|---|
| Right atrial pressure (mean) | 10 mm Hg | 0–6 mm Hg |
| Pulmonary artery pressure (S/D) | 24/12 mm Hg | 10–25/0–12 mm Hg |
| Pulmonary artery pressure (mean) | 18 mm Hg | 10–18 mm Hg |
| Pulmonary capillary wedge pressure (mean) | 12 mm Hg | 0–12 mm Hg |
| Blood pressure | 113/57 | |
| Mean arterial pressure | 76 mm Hg | 70–90 mm Hg |
| Cardiac output | 6.72 liters/min | 4–8 liters/min |
| Cardiac index | 2.8 liters/min/m$^2$ | 2.5–4 liters/min/m$^2$ |
| Heart rate | 97 beats/min | |
| Stroke index | 28.9 ml/beat/m$^2$ | 35–70 ml/beat/m$^2$ |
| Systemic vascular resistance | 785.7 dyne-sec/cm$^{-5}$ | 950–1,300 dyne-sec/cm$^{-5}$ |

intubated when he returned to the intensive care unit and was placed on an Emerson volume ventilator with the following settings: fraction of inspired oxygen ($FiO_2$), 40 percent; tidal volume, 10 ml/kg; respiration rate, 10 breaths/min; and positive end expiratory pressure (PEEP), 5 cm $H_2O$. Bilateral breath sounds were clear to auscultation. His color was pink with good capillary refill. The Swan-Ganz catheter and an arterial line were connected to transducers for continuous monitoring; blood return and waveforms were satisfactory. Two atrial pacing wires were connected to an atrial pacer at 7 mA, rate 80 for underlying sinus bradycardia at 50 beats/min. Two pericardial chest tubes connected to a chest drainage unit showed small amounts of bloody drainage. Pedal pulses were weak. His rectal temperature was 34°C. Mr. S's hemodynamic profile at this time indicated that afterload reduction would be helpful (Table 8–3). He was started on sodium nitroprusside (Nipride), which was increased gradually to 0.3 μg/kg/min with improvement in cardiac index.

Five hours postoperatively, Mr. S was awake, moving all extremities to command. His temperature had returned to normal. Because his heart rate had increased to a sinus rate of 85 beats/min, the atrial pacer was discontinued. The Nipride infusion was also gradually discontinued. His urine output remained excellent until his pulmonary capillary wedge pressure dropped to nearly 9 mm Hg. His hematocrit was 30 percent at this time, so 2 units packed red blood cells were administered; this

**Table 8–3** Mr. S: Postsurgical Hemodynamic Profiles

| Parameter | 11:15 | 12:55 | Time 16:22 | 0400 |
|---|---|---|---|---|
| Temperature (°C) | 34.8 | 35.8 | 37.9 | 38.1 |
| Heart rate (beats/min) | 80 | 80 | 85 | 95 |
| Blood pressure | 120/67 | 123/71 | 126/68 | 109/56 |
| Mean arterial pressure (mm Hg) | 83 | 86 | 83 | 73 |
| Pulmonary artery pressure | 25/15 | 27/21 | 28/20 | 24/10 |
| Pulmonary artery (mean) pressure | 19 | 21 | 20 | 16 |
| Pulmonary capillary wedge pressure (mm Hg) | 19 | 17 | 10–12 | 9 |
| Right atrial pressure (mm Hg) | 10 | 9 | 8 | 6 |
| Cardiac output (liters/min) | 4.38 | 5.15 | 5.52 | 5.63 |
| Cardiac index (liters/min/m²) | 1.84 | 2.17 | 2.32 | 2.37 |
| Systemic vascular resistance (dyne-sec/cm$^{-5}$) | 1,332 | 1,197 | 1,086 | 953 |
| Nipride infusion (μg/kg/min) | 0.15 | 0.30 | Off | Off |
| Volume | None | None | 2 units packed red blood cells | 250 ml hespan |

**Table 8–4** Nursing Care Plan: Cardiac Surgery after Acute Myocardial Infarction

| Patient Problem | Patient Goals | Target Date | Nursing Actions |
|---|---|---|---|
| Potential decreased cardiac output related to cardiac surgical procedure | The patient will maintain adequate output as evidenced by | Date of surgery | The nurse will |
| | • hemodynamic parameters within normal limits | | • observe and document ECG |
| |    • heart rate $> 60 < 110$ | | • set bedside alarms for heart rate, mean arterial pressure, and left atrial pressure |
| |    • blood pressure systolic $> 90 < 150$ mm Hg | | • zero and calibrate hemodynamic monitoring lines every 4 hours and record pressures as ordered |
| |    • mean arterial pressure $> 60 < 110$ mm Hg | | • record cuff blood pressure every shift |
| |    • left atrial pressure $> 5 < 12$–$14$ mm Hg | | • evaluate and record vital signs and pedal pulses as ordered |
| |    • cardiac index $> 2.5$ liters/min/m$^2$ | | • record chest drainage every 1 hour; milk chest tubes prior to recording; turn patient side to side to facilitate drainage |
| | • Color and perfusion adequate | | • draw blood sample and evaluate activated clotting time if chest drainage $> 200$ ml first hour; administer protamine IV slowly if indicated |
| |    • pedal pulses $> + 2$ | | |
| |    • skin pink and warm | | • record urine output every 1 hour |
| | • postoperative bleeding adequately controlled: chest tube drainage $< 100$ ml/hour with no other bleeding sites | | • give fluids and/or vasodilators to keep mean arterial and left atrial pressures within desired limits; calculate systemic vascular resistance as necessary to guide vasodilator administration |
| | • renal function adequate: urine output $> 20$–$30$ ml/hour | | |

**Table 8–4** continued

| Patient Problem | Patient Goals | Target Date | Nursing Actions |
|---|---|---|---|
| | | | • order potassium level determination immediately and every 4 hours; give potassium chloride replacement as necessary to keep potassium 3.5–4.5 mEq/liter |
| | | | • atrially pace at 80–90 beats/min for sinus bradycardia; discontinue pacing if heart rate > 80 beats/min |
| | | | • facilitate warming by |
| | | | • using blood warmer |
| | | | • keeping patient covered with warm blankets while hypothermic |
| Respiratory insufficiency related to decreased level of consciousness resulting from anesthesia | The patient will experience no respiratory insufficiency as evidenced by | | The nurse will |
| | • arterial blood gases within normal limits | | • observe and document respiration rate and quality, auscultate every 1 hour and whenever necessary |
| | • $Pao_2 > 80$ mm Hg | | • observe for readiness to wean from ventilator as evidenced by the patient's |
| | • $Paco_2 < 45 > 35$ mm Hg | | • responding to verbal stimuli appropriately |
| | • pH > 7.35 < 7.50 | | • triggering ventilator or breathing between intermittent mandatory ventilation breaths |
| | • patient-initiated breathing | | |
| | • tidal volume > 5 ml/kg | | • being able to lift head |
| | • vital capacity > 12 ml/kg | | • begin weaning after measuring negative inspired force, tidal volume, |
| | • respiratory rate < 22 breaths/min | | |
| | • negative inspired force > 30 cm $H_2O$ | | |
| | • lungs clear to auscultation | | |
| | • adequate cough | | |

and vital capacity and ensuring that they are within normal limits

- evaluate arterial blood gases after each ventilator change
- suction on return from operating room and every 2 hours or whenever necessary
- observe and record quality of endotracheal secretions
- turn patient side to side every 2 hours
- insert nasogastric tube for drainage to decrease abdominal pressure and facilitate lung expansion

The nurse will

- measure temperature continuously for 24 hours; then every 4 hours
- clean all incisions and IV sites daily, starting 18 hours after surgery, using peroxide and povidone-iodine (Betadine) daily
- change IV tubing and bottles every 24 hours
- culture any purulent drainage
- encourage early ambulation, coughing, and deep breathing
- observe and record nature of endotracheal secretions; culture foul-smelling secretions

Discharge date

Impaired skin integrity related to surgical sites, hemodynamic lines, IV sites, Foley catheter, and endotracheal tube

The patient will display no signs of infection as evidenced by

- temperature < 38°C
- no swelling, redness, edema or purulent drainage from
  - surgical wounds
  - IV sites
  - hemodynamic lines
  - clear urine output
- endotracheal secretions clear to white without foul smell

elevated the pulmonary capillary wedge pressure to 12 mm Hg. Urine output increased to acceptable levels after volume infusion.

On postoperative day 1, Mr. S was stable, awake, with normal arterial blood gas levels on 40 percent T piece. During this time, his pulmonary capillary wedge pressure decreased to 9 mm Hg, urine output was less than 30 ml/hour for 2 consecutive hours, and hematocrit was 32 percent. Mr. S was given 250 ml hespan, which improved his urine output and cardiac index.

He was extubated without difficulty and was able to cough well with help. His lungs were clear in the upper lobes with bibasilar rales that cleared with coughing. Chest tubes were removed, as was the Swan-Ganz catheter, arterial line, and peripheral intravenous line.

The postoperative ECG continued to show Q waves in leads $V_1$ through $V_3$. Postoperative laboratory results were acceptable, and Mr. S was transferred from the intensive care unit without difficulty. He ambulated that evening and progressed in activity over the next 5 days to walking approximately 1 mile. Discharge instruction, which covered diet, exercise, and incisional care, began on postoperative day 3. On postoperative day 7, his atrial and ventricular pacing wires were discontinued without complications, and he was discharged home with a home walking program.

He returned to his cardiologist's office after 1 month and was discharged to return to work and enter the cardiac rehabilitation program.

Mr. S is representative of many patients who experience AMI today. Streptokinase infusions have become relatively commonplace in the initial treatment of AMI, but they do not lyse the underlying coronary artery lesion. Many times, the stenosis requires further treatment to establish an optimal blood flow to that portion of the myocardium. Because Mr. S had few complications during his treatment, his case study provides information that can be used in caring for many cardiac surgical patients.

## NURSING CARE PLAN

The nursing care plan designed for Mr. S addresses the most critical components in the care of the cardiac surgical client (Table 8–4). Although there are numerous methods for monitoring preload and afterload in cardiac surgical clients, the principles and goals of therapy remain the same.

**NOTES**

1. W.E. Walker et al., "Streptokinase Reperfusion and Early Surgical Revascularization in Patients with Acute Myocardial Infarction," *Southern Medical Journal* 75 (1982): 1531–1537.

2. P.L. Whitlow et al., "Enhancement of Left Ventricular Function by Glucose-Insulin-Potassium Infusion in Acute Myocardial Infarction," *American Journal of Cardiology* 49 (1982): 811.

3. M.A. DeWood et al., "Intra-aortic Balloon Counterpulsation with and without Reperfusion for Myocardial Infarction Shock," *Circulation* 61 (1980): 1105.

4. E. Zeitler, A.R. Gruntzig, and W. Schoop, "Percutaneous Vascular Recanalization," Berlin, Springer-Verlag, 1978.

5. A.R. Gruntzig, A. Senning, and W.E. Siegenthaler, "Non-operative Dilatation of Coronary Artery Stenosis: Percutaneous Transluminal Coronary Angioplasty," *New England Journal of Medicine* 301 (1979): 61.

6. R.I. Levy et al., "Percutaneous Transluminal Coronary Angioplasty—A Status Report," *New England Journal of Medicine* 305 (1981): 399.

7. B.J. Messmer, W. Merx, J. Meyer, P. Bardos, C. Minale, and S. Effert. "New Developments in Med/Surg Treatment of AMI," *Annals of Thoracic Surgery* 35 (1983): 70–78.

8. J.E. Markis, M. Malagold, J.A. Parker, et al., "Myocardial Salvage after Intracoronary Thrombolysis with Streptokinase in Acute Myocardial Infarction," *New England Journal of Medicine* 305 (1981): 777–782.

9. J.F. Spann et al., "High-dose, Brief Intravenous Streptokinase Early in Acute MI," *American Heart Journal* 104 (1982): 939.

10. R. Schroder et al., "Intravenous Short-term Infusion of Streptokinase in Acute MI," *Circulation* 67 no. 3 (1983): 536–548.

11. E.H. Levine, H.K. Cold, R.C. Linback, W. Daggett, W.G. Austen, and M.J. Buckley: "Safe Early Revascularization after Acute MI," *Circulation* 60, suppl 1 (1979): 5–9.

12. E.L. Jones, T.F. Waites, J.M. Craver, J.M. Bradford, J.S. Douglas, S.B. King, D.K. Bone, E.R. Dorney, S.D. Clements, T. Thompkins, and C.R. Hacher, "Coronary Bypass for Relief of Persistent Pain following Acute MI," *Annals of Thoracic Surgery* 32 (1981): 33–34.

13. R.P. Greenwald, quoted in D.L. Nunnely, G.L. Grunkemeier, J.F. Teply, P.A. Abbruzzese, J.S. Davis, S. Khonsare, and A. Starr, "Coronary Bypass Operation following Acute Complicated MI," *Journal of Thoracic and Cardiovascular Surgery* 85 (1983): 485–491.

14. R. Berg, S.L. Selinger, J.L. Leonard, R.P. Greenwald, and W.P. O'Grady, "Immediate CAB for Acute Evolving MI," *Journal of Thoracic and Cardiovascular Surgery* 81 (1981): 493–497.

15. S.S. Phillips, C. Kongthahworn, R.H. Zeff, M. Benson, L. Ianione, T. Brown, and D.F. Gordon, "Emergency Coronary Artery Revascularization: A Possible Therapy for AMI," *Circulation* 60 (1979): 241–246.

16. M. DeWood, J. Spores, R. Notske, H. Lang, J. Shields, C. Simpson, L. Rudy, and R. Grunwald: "Medical and Surgical Treatment of MI," *American Journal of Cardiology* 44 (1979): 1356–1364.

# Appendixes

# Nursing Research Questions Regarding Hemodynamic Monitoring

Delphi Study Question No. 10

What are the effects of patient positioning on cardiovascular and pulmonary functioning of various types of critically ill patients?

Delphi Study Question No. 12

What nursing measures . . . are most effective in preventing infections
in patients with invasive lines and/or undergoing invasive procedures?

*Source: 1982 Compilation of Research Abstracts for Critical Care Nurses—A Review of AACN Delphi Study Topics* by S. Dunbar (Ed.), pp. 29 and 37, American Association of Critical-Care Nurses, © 1984.

# Standards to Consult in Developing Nursing Policies/ Procedures Related to Hemodynamic Monitoring

*Carolyn Chalkley, R.N., M.S.N.*

Nursing Process

- AACN Process Standards I, II, III, IV, V
- JCAH Nursing Service Standard IV

Management

- AACN Structure Standards VI, VII, VIII, IX, X, XI
- JCAH Nursing Service Standards II, III, VI, VII
- JCAH Special Care Units Standards II, IV

Safety

- JCAH Special Care Units Standards V, VII
- JCAH Plant, Technology and Safety Management Standards IX, X, XI, XII
- AACN Structure Standards I, II, III, IV, V

Infection Control

- JCAH Infection Control Standard III
- AACN Structure Standard V

Education

- JCAH Nursing Service Standard V
- JCAH Special Care Units Standard III
- AACN Structure Standard VIII

*Key: AACN*, American Association of Critical-Care Nurses; *JCAH*, Joint Commission on the Accreditation of Hospitals

# Sample Standards of Nursing Practice Related to Hemodynamic Monitoring

*Charmaine Frederick, R.N., B.S.N., C.C.R.N.*

Standard I
The critical care nurse will demonstrate knowledge of cardiovascular anatomy and physiology and their physical assessment.

Standard II
The critical care nurse will coordinate the assembly of equipment necessary for insertion of monitoring devices.

Standard III
The critical care nurse will obtain hemodynamic measurements accurately and correlate them with physical assessment findings.

Standard IV
The critical care nurse will be able to identify selected cardiovascular pathologic conditions by interpreting waveforms.

Standard V
The critical care nurse will recognize measurement problems, correct them, and/or seek a physician's intervention.

Standard VI
The critical care nurse will make appropriate interventions based on hemodynamic data.

Standard VII
The critical care nurse will recognize complications associated with invasive monitoring catheters.

Standard VIII
The critical care nurse will discontinue the use of catheters when ordered.

# Factors to Consider in the Evaluation and Purchase of Bedside Hemodynamic Equipment

*Charmaine Frederick, R.N., B.S.N., C.C.R.N.*
*Carolyn Chalkley, R.N., M.S.N.*

Functional Capabilities

- Twelve-lead electrocardiogram
- Total number of lines displayed on scope
- Total number of pressure outlets and equal interchange for different sources of pressure
- Temperature modes, respiration rate, apnea detection
- Synchronization with intra-aortic balloon pumping and cardioversion
- Size and visibility range of bedside and central display screens
- Printouts (dual channel, calibrated)
- Memory, delay, cascade of screen display
- Alarm selection, event detection, arrhythmia diagnosis
- Obliteration of respiratory motion for pressure measurements

Data Management Capabilities

- Bedside entry of patient data
- Trending and calculation packages
- Hard copy printouts

Expansion Capabilities (e.g., remote terminals for physician access)
Adaptability with Current Accessories, Supplies, and Computer Systems
Preventive and Reparative Maintenance
Reusable Accessories/Supplies

- Reprocessing
- Sterilization/cleaning procedures

- Nursing time
- Technical support time

Disposable Accessories/Supplies

- Cost per unit
- Quantity to be ordered/stored
- Shipment time
- Shelf life
- Storage space
- Reimbursement
- Compatibility with reusable accessories/supplies

Service Record and Financial Statement of Vendor(s)
Vendor Contract

- Availability of service personnel
- Backup equipment
- In-service materials
- Training plan and resource personnel for staff (e.g., medical, biomedical, nursing)
- Replacement discounting
- Future purchase discounting
- Automatic updating of purchased equipment

Environmental Compatibility/Restructure

# Index

## A

Acetylcholine, 53
Actin filaments, 5, 6, 24–26, 32
Action potential, 23–24, 43
Active hyperemia, 54
Acute myocardial infarction (AMI), 169–170. *See also* Cardiac surgery case study
Adult respiratory distress syndrome (ARDS)
  management, 148–151, 155
  monitoring, 146–148
  nursing care plan, 152–155
  overview, 145–146
Afterload, 32–34, 40, 73, 173
Aminophylline, 150
Anatomy
  cardiac cells, 3, 5–6
  cardiac wall, 6–8
  chambers, 11–13
  conduction system, 17–19
  great vessels, 12, 13
  heart structure, 3
  peripheral vasculature, 19–22
  valves, 8–11
  vasculature, 14–17
Anrep effect, 35
Anterior descending artery, 15–16
Antishock pants, 109
Aorta, 13
Aortic pressure, 70, 73–75
Arterial pressures, 34, 73–76, 98, 162

Arteries, 12–16, 19–20, 22
Arterioles, 20, 22, 52
Atria, 11–13
Atrial dysrhythmias, 93
Atrial electrogram, 69
Atrial flutter, 94
Atrial pressures, 37, 76–80, 122
Atrial systole, 29, 69
Atrioventricular bundle, 19
Atrioventricular node, 18–19, 41
Atrioventricular valves, 8–10, 30
Autonomic nervous system, 41–43, 53, 61, 63, 64, 97, 132
Autoregulation, 31–32, 35, 40, 54

## B

Bacteremia, 131
Bainbridge reflex, 42–43
Baroreceptors, 55, 64
$\beta$-blockers, 169
Bipolar atrial electrogram, 69
Blood flow, 52–54
Blood pressure regulation
  arteries, 54–56
  capacitance vessels, 59
  exchange vessels, 57–59
  hypertension and, 102
  pulmonary vessels, 59–62
Blood volume, 94–96
Body temperature, 43
Bronchial arteries, 12